IMPORTANT NOTES TO MY READERS:

these pages, I have some updated information to share with you... Shortly after its release, this book became unavailable due to a publishing contract I had. While the book was out of print, I fretted that the world was missing the best way to bake grain free and paleo goodies! What makes these recipes so different from others is the addition of whole foods that blend in combination with the flours, truly making a cupcake with a traditional taste and texture <u>without</u> **the use of extracted, high glycemic starches.**

Most importantly: Over this time period I discovered these recipes could also easily be made in the blender, so the food processor is no longer a requirement. Both almond and coconut flours have become less expensive and more readily available, so by using the chart on page 36 you can substitute almond and coconut flour for the blanched almonds and shredded coconut. The recipe directions in this book are for the food processor, so **to use your blender simply follow the directions on the next page.**

When my publishing company was bought by another publishing company, it created great contract delays, however, I'm happy to say that another book is now in the works. My passion has expanded to baking breads and other goods (which we now sell online and to the food service industry).

Why I don't use Cassava Flour... many of you know that cassava is the ground flour of the yuca (or manioc) root, the same root that tapioca starch is derived from. While processing and cooking eliminates the toxic levels of cyanide that is present in this root, it is poisonous in its natural state, so I opt to leave it out of my family's food. Japan doesn't even allow it to be used as a human food source. It's currently becoming popular to many paleo enthusiasts as a grain free alternative flour, but I urge my friends to consider choices such as real foods like sweet potato or plantain, both available in flour form.

No food processor? No problem!
NEW! Blender Directions...

1. Position your oven rack to the middle portion of oven.
2. Preheat the oven to 350°F.
3. Line muffin pan with 12 cupcake paper liners and set aside.
4. Use the chart on page 36 to substitute the blanched almonds and shredded coconut for **blanched** almond *flour* and organic coconut *flour*.
5. In a medium-sized bowl, sift together the dry ingredients and set aside.
6. In your blender, blend together the wet ingredients until smooth.
7. Pour the wet ingredients into the dry and whisk to combine. The batter should be like thick pancake batter, so whisk in a little more almond or coconut flour if the batter is too loose.
8. Fill the cupcake liners about 2/3 full.
9. Bake about 30 minutes until the tops are firm and spring back when touched.
10. Cover with aluminum foil if they begin to brown.

NOTE: the 'Wet' Ingredients include the eggs and whatever the raw, chopped, whole food is (zucchini, beet, etc) and any extracts, lemon juice, etc.

California Country Gal's
Sweet secretS

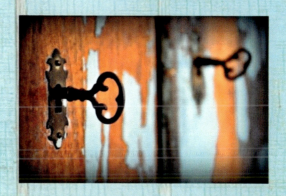

Annabelle Lee

Paleo Friendly   Low Glycemic   Guilt Free & Delicious

Real Food CUPCAKES!

Beyond GRAIN FREE *Beyond* GLUTEN FREE *Beyond* DIETING!

Photography by Jacob Lee and Derek Hackett

a California Country Gal's

SWEET SECRETS

Copyright © 2013-2018 by Annabelle Lee | CCG, Inc.
Photographs Copyright © 2013-2018 by Annabelle Lee | CCG, Inc.

All rights reserved.
No part of this publication may be reproduced, stored in a retrieval system, or transmitted, in any form or by any means, electronic, mechanical, photocopying, recording, or otherwise, without the prior written permission of the author.

Published by CCG, Inc.
For information please email hello@californiacountrygal.com.

www.californiacountrygal.com

Library of Congress Cataloging-in-Publication Data

Please Note: The information in this book is true and complete to the best of our knowledge. This book is intended only as an information guide for those wishing to know more about baking with real whole foods and the health related benefits. In no way is this book intended to replace, countermand, or conflict with the advice given to you by your own physician. The ultimate decision concerning care should be made between you and your physician. We strongly recommend you follow your decisions with the assistance of his or her advice. Information in this ebook is general and is offered with no guarantees on the part of the author. The author and publisher expressly disclaim responsibility for any adverse effects that may result in the use or application of the recipes or information contained in this book.

ISBN-13: 978-1481226554

Cover and Interior design by A&T Teamworks

Photography by Jacob Lee and Derek Hackett

10 9 8 7 6 5 4 3 2 1

First Edition 2013
Second Edition 2016
Third Edition 2018

"I've seen many lives elevated – renewed and healed – through the power of wholesome nutritious food…Because of its healing potential and spiritual energy, food should be sacred to us – prepared with reverence and consumed with gratitude. But alas, even though the passing decades have brought us more insight and wisdom, many of us still make our food choices based on…our desire for immediate gratification."

The Baby Boomer Diet – 2011 - Donna Gates of Body Ecology
Nutritional Consultant, Author, and Lecturer

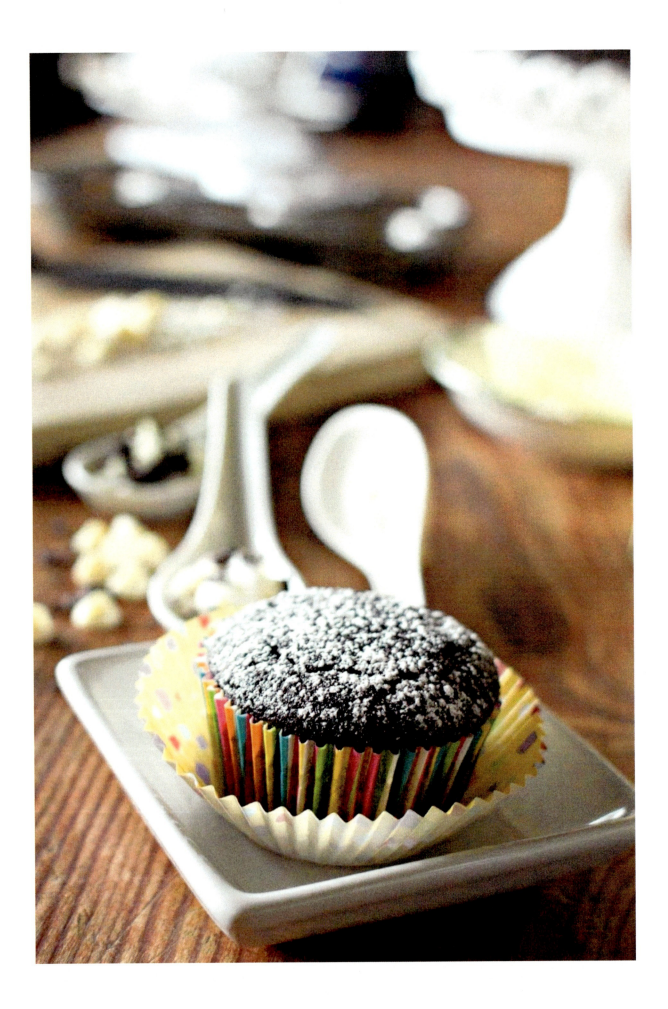

I Dedicate this Book to YOU

Thank you so much for taking the time to read and share this book!

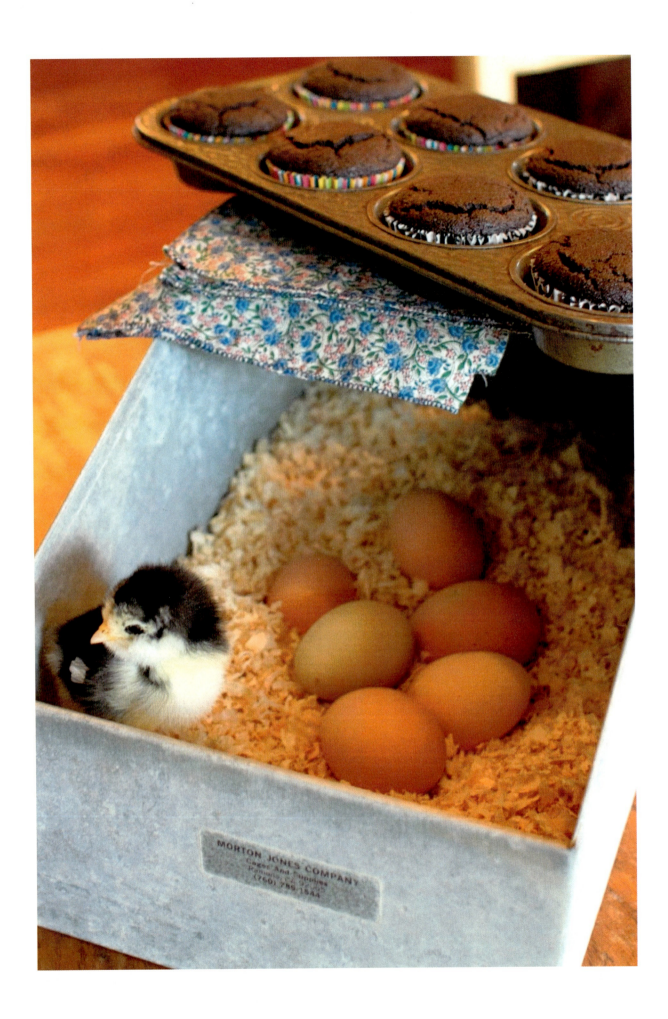

Contents

DEDICATION

INTRODUCTION   3
    Just Eat Real Whole Foods   4
    Keeping It Simple   6

BAKE WITH LOVE…EAT and BE VIBRANT   8
    Getting Wise to Whole Food NON-Ingredients   8
        Bad Fats & Oils   8
        Wheat & Grains   10
        Milk   11
        Sugar   12
    About Whole Food Baking INGREDIENTS   15
        Why These Ingredients?   16
        Other Ingredients   25
    About Sweeteners   27
        Sweeteners used in this Book   27
        Other Sweeteners   30

GET READY TO BAKE and BE SURPRISED   33
    Real Whole Food Baking EQUIPMENT   33
    Helpful TIPS   33
    Conversions & Equivalents   36

THE RECIPES
    CUPCAKES   39
    FROSTINGS   105

INGREDIENT RESOURCES   123
RESOURCES   124
INDEX

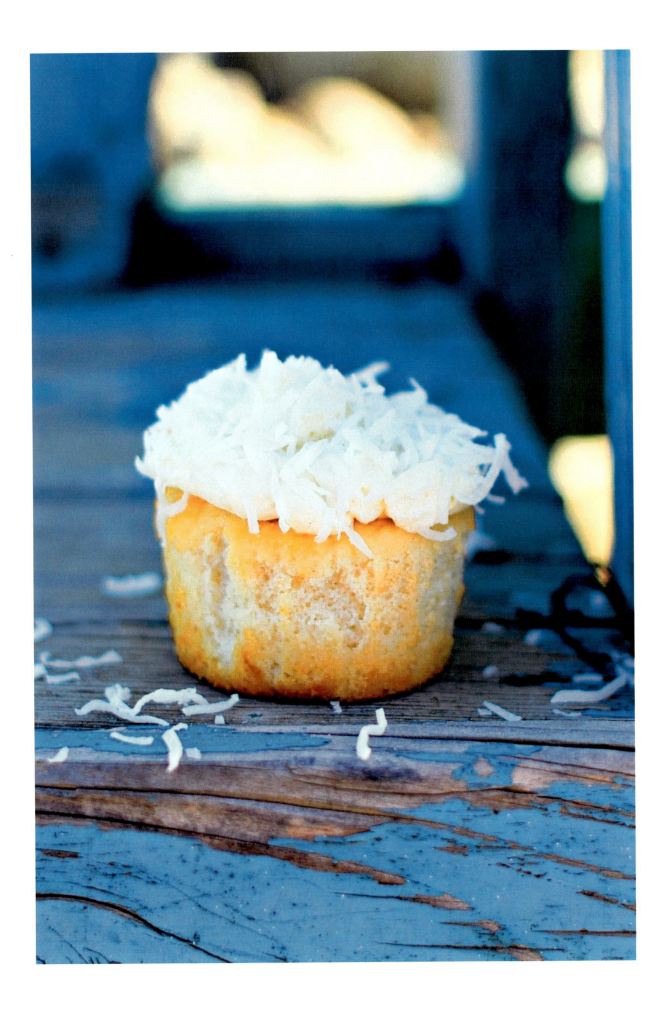

"People have lived and thrived on high-protein, high-fat diets; on low-protein, high-carb diets; on diets high in raw milk and cream; even on diets high in animal blood (the Masai). And they've done so without the ravages of degenerative diseases that are epidemic in modern life…Here's what they haven't done: thrived on food with bar codes."
Jonny Bowden, PhD, Author and Lecturer

Introduction

Years ago, I embarked on a path to help relieve what doctors labeled as 'auto-imune' symptoms. I found that by omitting certain 'foods' and increasing my consumption of whole plant foods my symptoms improved. I have now come to believe that most 'auto-immune disease' is brought on by chronic, stealth infections and that our bodies need optimal nutrients in order to subdue these invaders and begin to heal. Today, we have 'new' diseases running rampant. Funny how there seems to be a 'pill' for everything, but there rarely seems to be a 'cure'. We have epidemic proportions of obesity, diabetes, autism, ADHD, bi-polar disorder, allergies, Alzheimer's, fatty liver, heart disease, bowel disease, fibromyalgia, osteoporosis, cancer and pharmaceutical addictions. There's confusion and disagreement amongst scientists and medical professionals as to how and why we get them. **Dietary beliefs are at the forefront yet seem to be more hotly debated than ever before.**

With the end of World War II, sugar rationing ended. Sugar and wheat flour were the cheapest ingredients that could be put in virtually *everything* and be made to taste like just about *anything*. They also happen to be addictive and they are still used abundantly in virtually all our packaged and pre-made 'foods'.

The most recent studies report that **high blood sugar, vitamin D deficiency** (weren't we told to stay out of the sun, *our source of vitamin D*, and to slather on that chemical sunscreen?) **and lack of physical exercise are the** *three most prevalent determining factors of cancer patients.* SUGAR KILLS. Wheat flour and extracted starches, such as those used abundantly in gluten-free baking (corn, potato, tapioca, arrowroot, rice, etc.) break down in our bodies and turn to sugar as quickly as eating table sugar. *Now, think about what you're doing when you combine refined flours with sugar and/or starch for baking. You're doubling and tripling your trouble!*

To make matters worse, 60 or so years of antibiotic use in humans and livestock has left us in a weakened, imbalanced state, allowing the overgrowth of dangerous yeasts and bacteria, which thrive on starchy, simple carbohydrates and sugar. These pathogenic microbes can destroy the balance of our **digestive tract, *the lifeline of our body*,** even allowing dangerous microbes to enter our bloodstreams causing 'mystery/auto-immune' diseases. More predominate with each generation, we have passed down this imbalanced microflora and weakened immune system to our children and we *honestly wonder why so many suffer from gut issues?* Or, why gut issues are a symptom of so many 'syndromes' and 'diseases' (autism, for instance)? Our beneficial bacteria continually create essential nutrients, antioxidants and anti-inflammatory compounds that keep us strong and healthy. **The latest research is now connecting the types and amounts of flora in our guts with virtually all of our major diseases, including obesity.**

Why do you suppose the two most common food allergens, wheat and dairy, have become the *base of the American diet?* Prior to the Age of Agriculture these items were not even part of the human diet. The proteins (gluten and casein) in these 'foods' share structural similarities with each other and are extremely difficult to digest. They also contain polypeptides that bind to our brains' morphine receptors like opiates. Do you know that convenience food manufacturers now routinely add gluten and casein to their products, often disguised under the label 'natural ingredients' *because* they are addicting? *If we are basically genetically predisposed to these substances through our grandparents' and parents' diets, and we pass this down to our children, and they to theirs, is it any wonder we have become a nation addicted to these 'foods' much like pharmaceutical pain killers?* Because our ancestors sought out ways to keep from going hungry, it doesn't mean filling up on grains makes the human body thrive.

JUST EAT REAL WHOLE FOODS

Which dietary guideline should we believe this year? Or, next year? Should we be Vegetarian, Vegan, Raw, Paleo or just Low Carb and Gluten-Free?

Contradicting all of these is our 'well-meaning' government preaching their 'food pyramid', right along with allowing chemical poisons and genetic modification into our 'food' supply, without so much as alerting us as to what we are buying or ingesting. No labeling (GMO's) and mislabeling (ingredients hidden under the word *Natural*, i.e.: high fructose corn syrup) WHY? Because it's all about Big Money. Virtually ALL of the big, money making crops today (wheat, corn, soy, cottonseed or canola oil, and even rice) are bred and cross-bred to increase yield and protein content and/or are genetically modified to withstand things like herbicides and pesticides and weather conditions. These are NOT the crops of yesteryear. **(And even if they were, does your best common sense tell you our diets should so heavily rely on wheat, corn and soy anyway????)**

Simply put, **Real Food** refers to foods that are grown or raised naturally and organically in nutrient-dense soils, preferably locally and in season, picked at the peak of their growth. It doesn't need to be ground or soaked or cooked to be edible. They're best prepared and eaten in ways that don't completely denature or devoid them of all of their life-giving nutrients, enzymes and naturally good micro-organisms. This means incorporating a higher percentage of raw foods into your meals by using quick and easy techniques (but these, my friends, are secrets for another book!).

Through the years, I've learned a lot by experimenting and what I've found works for me is NOT a strict, **ONE-WAY Diet Cult strategy.** It's not media hyped by our government and it's not how most of us learned to prepare food, and it's certainly a new way of baking... but, no worries, IT'S EASY! IT'S JUST BACK TO NATURE plus a couple of modern conveniences...the Food Processor and the Blender.

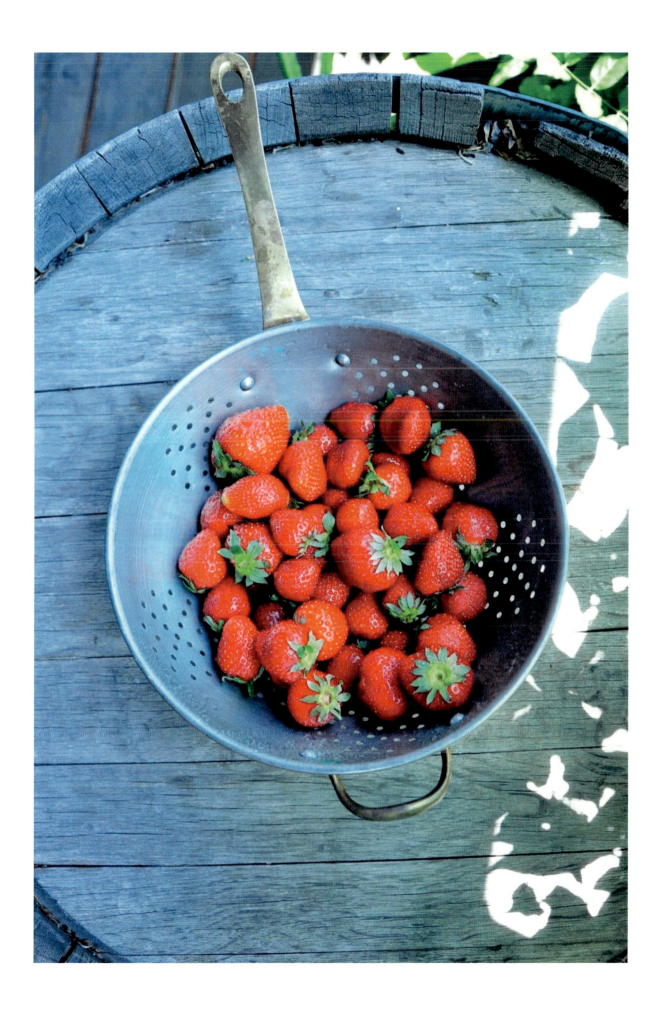

"The adoption of agriculture...can be viewed as a compromise in which convenience, societal evolution and food abundance were traded for health!"
2011 - Wheat Belly by Dr. William Davis – Bestselling Author

KEEPING IT SIMPLE

It's easy to fill up on convenience 'foods' these days, which doesn't leave much room to eat the quantity and quality of fresh fruits and veggies our bodies need to look and feel great. **That's why I add smoothies and juices to my day as well as keep a stash of my Real Food Cupcakes in the freezer.** If you make the time and space for a small garden, children especially love it when they learn the zucchini they helped grow in their garden is in their Cupcake!

Supplements are helpful, but real, whole, natural foods contain a multitude of vitamins, minerals, amino acids, enzymes, phytonutrients and all the other co-factors that **act in synergy** and as catalysts in any number of bodily functions and immune response.

Big Companies are using the words Organic and Gluten-Free as 'buzz words' now, just like they've done with the words 'Whole Grains' and 'Low Fat', enticing people to buy these products thinking they'll be eating healthy. **A product full of extracted starches, sugars, polyunsaturated oils and casein (used for flavorings and all sorts of things) and other hidden ingredients** *does not suddenly turn healthy because they've put 'gluten-free' or 'low-gat' on the label.*

While we're on the subject of *mislabeling*...**have you ever thought about what a** *Canola* **is, anyhow?** Well, now you'll know that it's the oil that's been extracted from the genetically modified Rapeseed plant, which, in its natural, unmodified state is naturally toxic to us.

*If you or someone you care for is ill with any disease, including Bi-Polar Disorder, ADHD, Auto-Immune Disorder, Allergies, etc, please look into a strict cleansing and healing diet such as the GAPS (Gut and Psychology Syndrome), SCD (Specific Carbohydrate Diet), or the Body Ecology (Candidiasis) Diet to enable your body to heal before adapting your own Real Whole Foods Lifestyle.

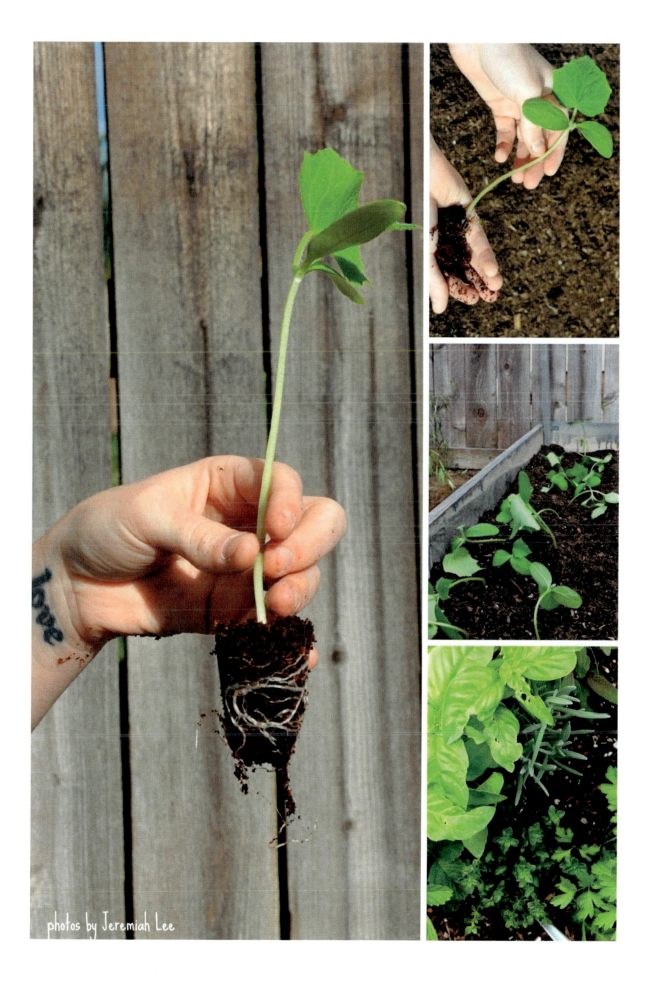

photos by Jeremiah Lee

"For the first generation of children in history that will live sicker and die younger than their parents. For their sakes and ours may we all work together to take back our health."
2012 - dedication by Dr. Mark Hyman in his most recent book, the Blood Sugar Solution.

BAKE with LOVE... EAT, and BE VIBRANT!

Now, I would like to share with you what I've learned through my years of seeking a simple, satisfying way to eat while feeling confident I'm helping my family get the proper nourishment to keep us out of the doctor's offices.

Raising four boys meant a lot of birthdays and other occasions where going without dessert (or a poor reproduction) was just not an option in my household. Cupcakes always seem to top my list: They're cute, versatile, quick, and easy and loved by just about everybody, right?! They've made a solid place for themselves in baking history, right between the cake and the cookie.

The Food Processors and Blenders on the market today make it EASIER THAN EVER to get the nutrients needed so that you can look, feel and BE VIBRANT! But the BEST NEWS is that you don't *EVER* have to feel like you're depriving yourself or your family because, when you're using these recipes, your baked goods will not just be packing a ton of nutrients but they'll be AMAZINGLY DELICIOUS!

GETTING WISE to *NON-FOOD* INGREDIENTS

BAD FATS/OILS... Just like we've been guided to 'eat more whole grains' and to 'stay out of the sun', for years now we've been told to eliminate saturated fats from our diet. Decades of completely wrong information has been promoted and severely damaged the health of generations of Americans. **Saturated fats are some of the healthiest fats we can eat.**

Man-made, mechanically hydrogenated, *fake* saturated fats should *never* be consumed. N*aturally* saturated fats in the form of butter, ghee (butter with milk solids removed), animal lard, coconut and palm oils are recognized and metabolized in our body in a natural and healthy way. Coconut oil is one of nature's rare sources of Lauric Acid, a medium-chain fatty acid which your body converts to energy. Its anti-microbial properties also help to keep yeast in check. **Saturated fats naturally hold all the hydrogen molecules they can and because of this they are 'stable' fats that can travel, intact through our bloodstream, escorting vitamins and minerals and other nutrients to various parts of our body. Saturated fats don't oxidize and breakdown in our body like the unstable polyunsaturated oils, such as corn and canola.**

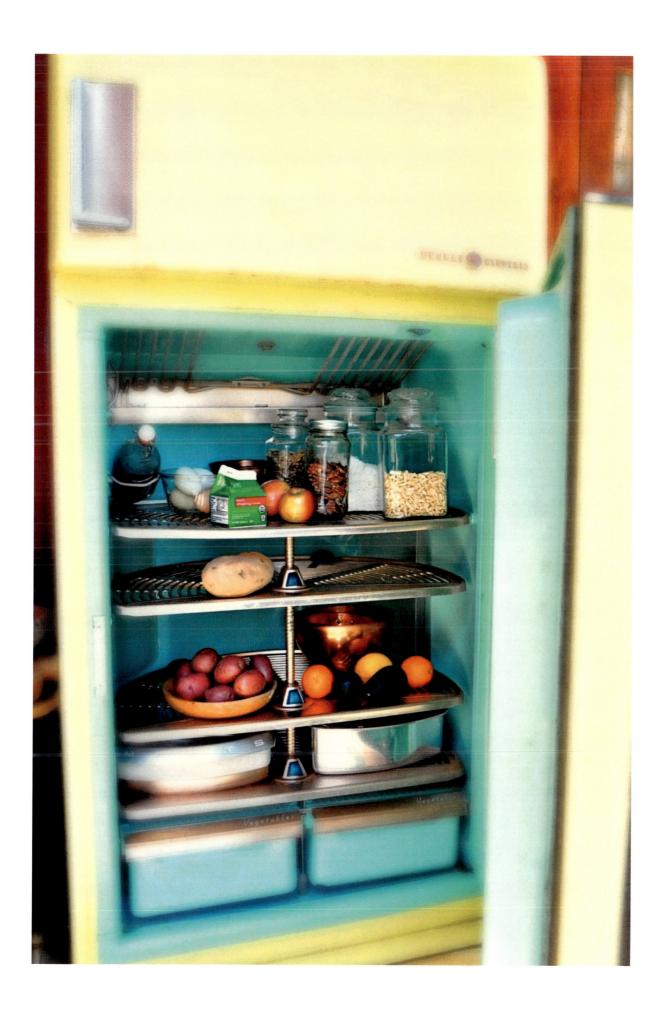

WHEAT... In the last 6 or 7 decades our modern wheat crops have been bred to withstand severe weather conditions, pathogens, insecticides and herbicides, as well as to increase its gluten content and per acre yield. **It has been used to 'feed the world', stave off hunger and to line the pockets of big agri-business, just like other crops such as soy and corn.**

According to a variety of scientific research; as well as Dr. Natasha Campbell, in her book 'Gut and Psychology Syndrome' and Dr. William Davis, in his bestseller 'Wheat Belly', wheat contains a specific complex carbohydrate that causes it to increase our glucose levels quicker than table sugar. **This means we're receiving a triple-weight-gaining-whammy when we're consuming all those baked goods or cereals containing the combination of wheat, starch, and sugar.**

What about 'whole grain' wheat? Well, have you heard of Agglutinin? Agglutinin is used by the plant to protect it from things like insects and fungi. Many plants have these lectins, which our bodies typically slough off, however Agglutinin is extremely difficult to break down. Research indicates it can attach to sugars and carbohydrates and cause them to clump together, hence the name Ag-**glu**-ti-nin. It's small enough to pass through cell membranes, intestinal walls and even cross the blood-brain barrier. *Apparently Agglutinin is in its highest concentration in the whole kernel.*

Besides, do you think we were REALLY meant to cross breed, spray with chemicles, harvest and grind up massive amounts of this inedible-in-its-natural-state 'food', and make it 80% of our diet? *Hmmmm, doesn't make much sense, does it?*

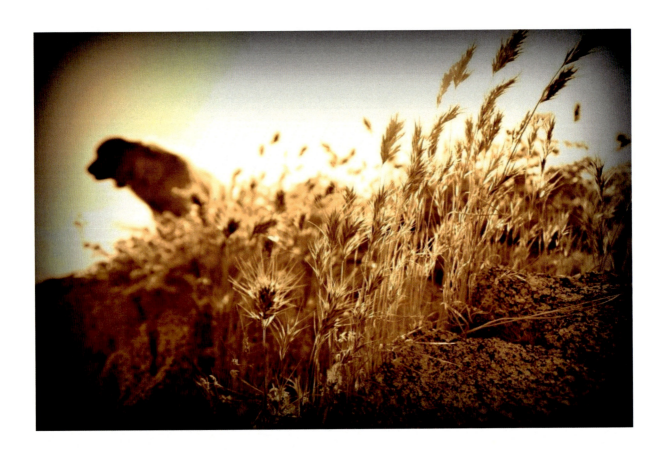

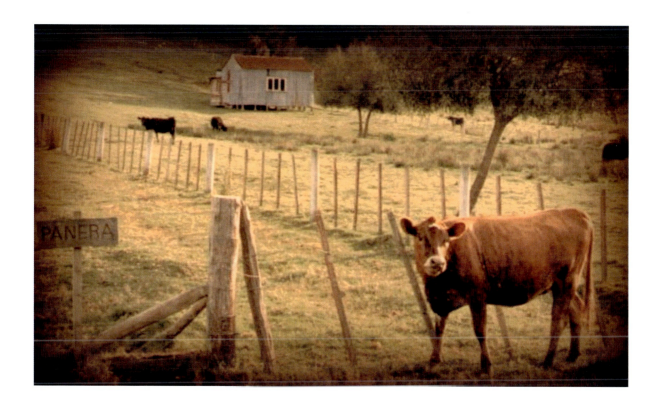

MILK... The casein protein in milk shares structural similarities to the gluten/gliaden protein in wheat and is difficult for humans to digest. Our American cattle are predominately the A1-type (big milk producers) which have a specific type of protein in their milk that's been linked with various health problems. **Unlike many other countries, *our American labeling system doesn't seem to think it's important to label the safer A2 beta-casein.***

No matter how much research confirms this, it will likely remain that way here in America; at least until 'Big Business' figures out a way to make more money from doing so. While our bodies may appear to have found their way to digest, utilize and store these substances as best it can, you must wonder about a skin condition, joint problem or headaches that may be resolved when these proteins are omitted.

So, happily, I can now tell you about HEAVY CREAM. Cream contains only a small amount of casein, and is usually well tolerated, even by those who can't drink milk products. Cream from Grass-fed Cows also supplies us the essential fatty acid, conjugated linoleic acid (CLA), which actually helps keep our cells from storing fat. *So, for these reasons and the fact that Cream is unsurpassed in taste and texture I enjoy it (organic and preferably raw) in a cup of coffee, sauces and in my desserts.* Butter, Sour Cream and Cream Cheeses are also on my happy list.

"When you take a bite of commercial food containing food additives, foreign chemicals enter your body whose safety was approved with 1930's knowledge."
2006 - The Hundred Year Lie - Randall Fitzgerald

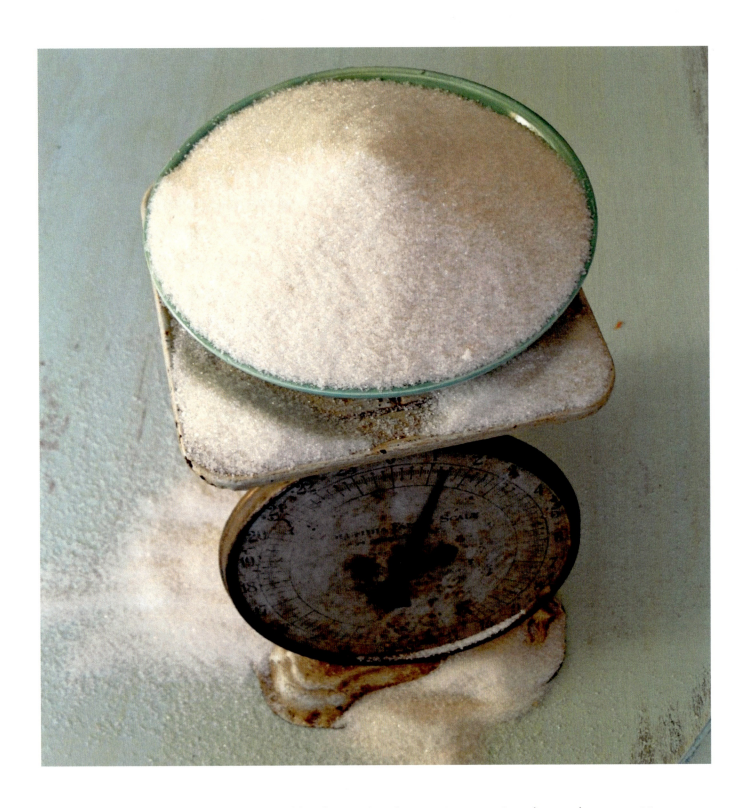

SUGAR... 2012 researchers linked high blood sugar levels to an increase in colorectal cancer. More recently they've discovered that many different cancer patients who consumed the most foods that produce high blood sugar had an 80% higher likelihood of dying during the 7-year study. A Korean study also confirmed higher death rates from cancer patients with higher blood sugar levels.

According to a newsletter by Dr. David Williams, a recent study from Australia has shown how high blood sugar levels cause shrinking in the parts of the brain connected with memory and emotion. This is just another example of the dangers of years of excess sugar and refined carbohydrates in our diet. **Sugar fluctuations become impossible for our bodies to control and cause age-related decline to the tune of researchers beginning to refer to Alzheimer's as type 3 diabetes.**

Baking our own goodies is a great start to allow us the opportunity to adjust the sweetness level down a notch or two and learn to use some of the healthier sweeteners we have available to us today. Fortunately, we now have several options to replace sugar safely and do not have to feel in the least bit deprived. My favorite choice for baking at the writing of this book is the fermented sugar alcohol Erythritol, which tastes great and travels safely through our digestive system.

While many manufacturers have begun to use the natural and safe sweeteners, Stevia and Monk Fruit, along with Erythritol, as I mentioned, they have hidden ingredients in their 'natural ingredient' list, so I still stay clear of them. You know that Coke used to contain cocaine back in the day, right? We seem to be repeating history…the names, faces and ingredients just keep changing. Because many companies hide things from consumers under 'natural ingredients' and 'natural flavors', allowing them to obtain a patent on their product, I prefer to buy a pure product from smaller companies and combine them in my recipes. **This also gives me more control of the flavor.**

STARCH… Maybe grandma used to treat you to tapioca pudding, or thicken her pies with it. Arrowroot, you might think it's good for you because so many healthy and gluten-free baking books use it instead of tapioca. Often these two are referred to as "flours" or "powders," but what they truly are is a pure starch, extracted from the root of the toxic cassava plant for tapioca or any number of different plants from around the world that is then labeled as "arrowroot." The starch is extracted in the same manner in which both corn and potato starch are extracted from those vegetables. Extracted starch is used for many things, including making glue, plastic, and stiffening shirt collars at the cleaners.

You may have heard about starch classified as 'resistant' starch being a beneficial prebiotic. Depending upon the food, the method of extraction and how it's prepared depends on how resistant to digestion it actually is. I encourage eating the whole food to obtain its benefits (which is why I use a lot of sweet potatoes). I talk more about resistant starch in the section on Sweet Potatoes. I don't believe we're meant to extract starch from its source and eat it, especially in large quantities. Plant foods with starch were meant to be eaten in their entirety so our bodies would obtain all of the compounds needed to properly digest and assimilate it. If we rely on starches to replace our beloved gluten in wheat, we are only jumping from the fire into the frying pan.

*"Our food choices are influenced by government subsidies
for agricultural mass production of poor-quality fats and sugars.
The government food pyramid reflects industry interests, not science".*
Life Extension Magazine - May 2013 - Dr. Mark Hyman, Bestselling Author

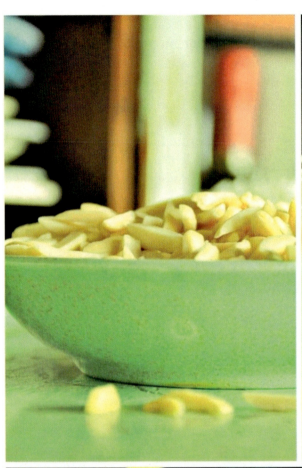
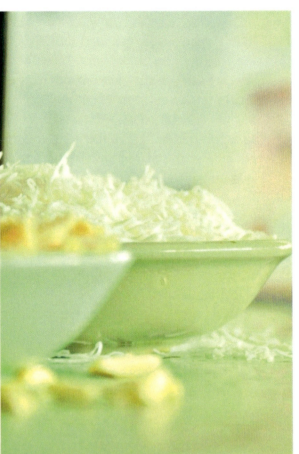
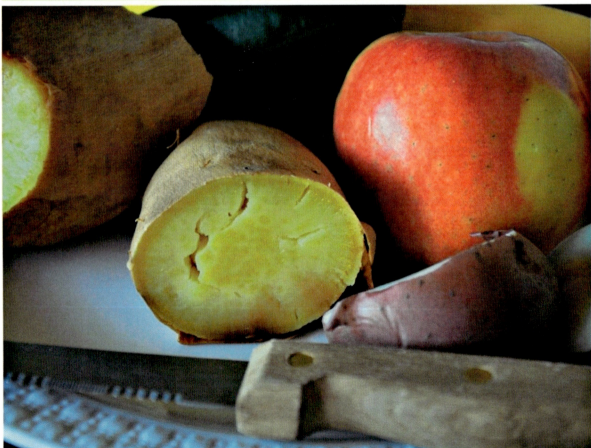

ABOUT WHOLE FOOD BAKING INGREDIENTS

Most of the ingredients I use should be quite easy for you to find. They're commonly used items that are **easy to grab** and will become your **'new staples'** *instead* of wheat or other grain/starchy flours, white sugar, milk and unstable oils. **Simply keep these ingredients on hand in your pantry, refrigerator or freezer!**

Remember, try your best to always buy Organic and preferably from Your Local Area Farms!

Coconut Flour, Erythritol, Palm Sugar and Palm Shortening are found in Natural Foods Stores, in the organic aisle of your supermarket and online if you prefer shopping that way. (See Resource page) **Note that we DON'T USE bean or grain flours or other typical, starchy gluten-free flours or blends.**

MAIN INGREDIENTS

Blanched Almonds or Almond Flour	Unsweetened Shredded Coconut	Eggs
Sweet Potatoes	Zucchini & Yellow Squash	Apples	Sea Salt
Walnuts Pecans	Red Skinned Potatoes	Erythritol	Palm Sugar

OTHER WHOLE FOODS USED

Pumpkin Bananas	Beets and Beet Greens	Baby Spinach	Avocados
Oranges Limes	Strawberries Cherries	Blueberries	Lemons

THE FROSTINGS

Palm Shortening	Heavy Cream/Coconut Cream	Cream Cheese	Butter
Mascarpone Cheese	Honey Maple Syrup	Freeze-dried Fruits	

ALSO USED

Coconut Flour   Cocoa   Egg White Powder   Baking Powder   Baking Soda   Stevia

OPTIONAL

Cream of Tartar   Guar Gum   Arrowroot

WHY THESE INGREDIENTS?

Not only are these 'Real Whole Foods' super nutritious, but I've found their flavors and textures blend together beautifully, making for delicious treats. Unbelievably healthy, and most with a high protein profile, they actually promote your body to burn fat by encouraging the production of glucagon, the 'weight-loss hormone'.

ALMONDS and other NUTS

The fruit of the Almond Tree is more accurately a seed than a nut, and many people that are sensitive to other nuts are able to eat Almonds. Nuts are full of vitamins, minerals and healthy fats. They've been linked to having positive affects in protecting human health in many ways; from cardiovascular disease to blood sugar levels, cancer and inflammatory disorders. The good fats in nuts also stimulate the production of a hormone that makes us feel full and even slows the emptying of the stomach.

Nuts also contain phytates and enzyme inhibitors which can bind minerals in the digestive tract and make digestion difficult. Grains, legumes, nuts, seeds, and even some innocent looking little sprouts can contain potent enzyme inhibitors which can cause an achy gut. For this reason, our ancestors learned that soaking the nuts in water for several hours leeches most of these compounds out into the water.

Why we use Blanched Almonds: Removing the skins by quickly blanching the almonds or buying blanched almonds, or ground, blanched almonds (almond 'flour') is beneficial in a few ways:

1. The highest concentration of these anti-nutrients is contained in the skin.
2. For that reason, I prefer using blanched almonds or almond flour rather than the meal (ground whole almonds, skin intact). They are also easier to bake with and taste delicious.
3. Long, hot storage of nuts, seeds and grains creates an environment for a very dangerous, cancer-causing fungi to grow, so most Almonds are pasteurized and irradiated now because of this issue; perhaps another good reason to remove the skins and to know where these items come from.

TIPS: If you buy whole almonds, you can blanch them yourself by immersing in boiling water for a minute; drain, cool and pop out of their skins. If you prefer Raw Almonds: for healthier, crunchy nuts soak them in warm water with a little Sea Salt for about 8 hours. Germinate them on a paper towel for about 12 hours, and then rub the skins off by rolling them in a kitchen towel. Dehydrate them in the oven at the lowest temperature setting with the door ajar.

A NOTE REGARDING OXALATES: Almonds, like many nuts and seeds contain oxalates. Oxalates are organic acids that our bodies use to create other substances. They are found in many great fruits and veggies, as well as some grains and legumes. Plants use them to protect themselves from bugs and infection.

Typically, oxalates are harmless because when a food is high in oxalates, healthy microflora in your intestines will metabolize them and any excess should bind with calcium in the intestines and then be escorted out of the body. When there's not enough calcium or if your gut has been damaged by antibiotics, wheat, or a sugary/starchy diet allowing yeast overgrowth, these oxalates can enter the bloodstream where they bind with calcium and may cause kidney stones or lodge in tissues or bones.

If oxalates concern you, you will want to make sure you are getting enough calcium and magnesium in your diet. You can also reduce the amount of oxalates in veggies that are high in them by boiling them and tossing the water. This may also work with almonds, which means using *blanched* almonds would be beneficial. **If you are among the small percentage of people who have trouble with oxalates, you may want to consider using Walnuts or another non-oxalate containing nut.**

While I mainly use Almonds for their light color, mild taste and moderate price, many other nuts can be used instead. *Blanched Almonds are typically more economical and easier to find than Almond Flour. When you need Almond Flour, it's quick and easy to grind your own Blanched Almonds.

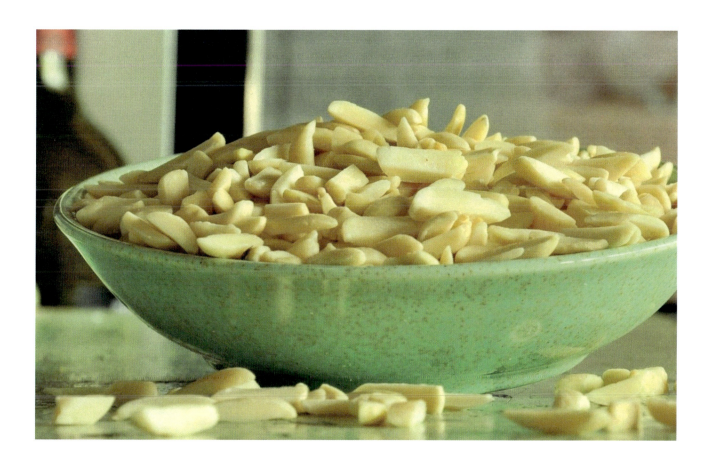

COCONUT

This wonderful fruit fell victim to the bad press of the evil *soy and cottonseed industry many years ago. Thankfully, newer research and media coverage has enlightened us! *For all those years the coconut was demonized, why do you suppose it still remained an ingredient in infant formula?* Seems like *someone* knew it was beneficial: its predominant fat is also found in human breast milk.

Coconuts are full of vitamins, minerals and many trace minerals. Extremely high in fiber with potent antimicrobial and antiviral qualities, coconut even helps strengthen our immune system. It is approximately 60% fat, and over 90% of it is saturated (*remember that's good!*) Its main fat, Lauric Acid, is a medium chain fatty acid that is quickly converted to energy by the liver, speeding up our metabolism and promoting a lean body!

Post WWII farmers tried to fatten their livestock using coconut oil, but failed miserably, reverting to soy and corn, with their slow-to-digest long-chain triglycerides, to fill that bill.

I much prefer using Whole, Shredded Coconut in my recipes as opposed to the now popular Coconut Flour because it isn't as highly processed and defatted so, as a 'whole food' it brings it's healthy, delicious oil with it.

Cultures who relied on the coconut as a staple in their diets were lean, healthy people. Some of these cultures even relied heavily on Taro, a very starchy root. Shortly after WWII, our American-made, sugar laden products made with both refined and hydrogenated oils and wheat became readily available. It was then that their healthy, virtually cancer and modern disease-free existence began to change.

*Cottonseeds and soybeans are thyroid suppressers and toxic in their natural state. Soy has been genetically modified and processed to make it edible. Ancient cultures knew to ferment it to create foods and condiments such as natto, tamari soy sauce, tempeh and miso before consuming it.

"The secret of the tropics:
The key to weight loss and vibrant health-is in eating the right kinds of fats,
avoiding refined carbohydrates, and consuming a diet of whole foods."
Cherie Calbom, MS and Bestselling Author of The Coconut Diet and The Complete Cancer Cleanse

EGGS

The nutrition contained within, as well as its numerous culinary uses, make eggs a favorite staple in my kitchen. Eggs contain all nine of the essential amino acids our body uses to make protein. If we're low in or missing just one of them, our bodies cannot make the other proteins it needs. **The yolk is a wonderful source of choline which is a nutrient vital to heart and brain function, as well as cell membrane health.**

Fresh and clean I often put them in smoothies and make meringues and eggnogs, thoroughly enjoying them in their raw form! *A raw egg from a healthy chicken raised in proper conditions does not pose a threat of contamination.* **Eggs should come from chickens that have been able to roam and enjoy feeding on plants and insects.** That's when you can enjoy their eggs containing the right balance of nutrients and Omega 3 oils rather than their less fortunate, grain-fed cousins, whose eggs pass on a highly unbalanced ratio of Omega 6 fatty acids.

So, plucking the eggs from my chickens' nests does not fill me with the same guilt as slaying Porky Pig. However, please consider researching the farm your eggs come from. Remember about mislabeling? Well, there are plenty of egg cartons that say they come from 'free range chickens' when in fact there's a little door open in a huge enclosed area, so that if the chicken ever finds it, it may get outside once.

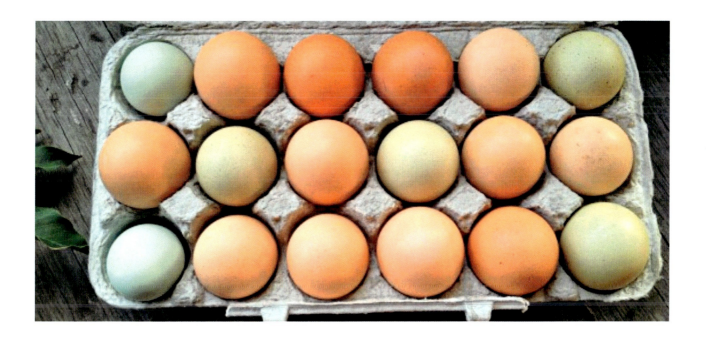

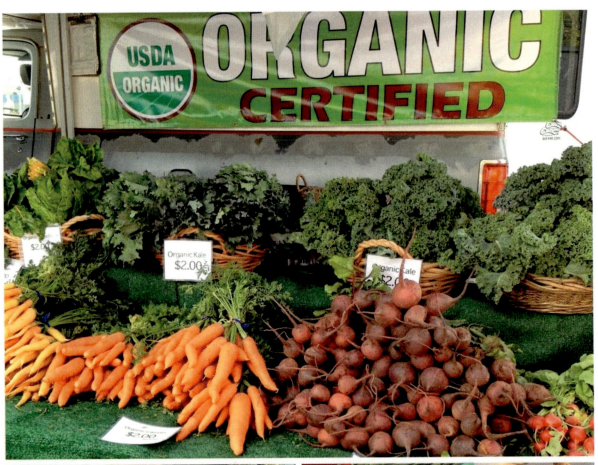
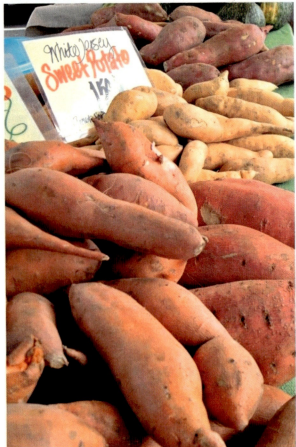
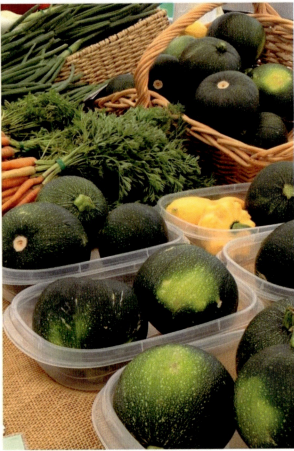

SWEET POTATOES and YAMS

Do you know that sweet potatoes and yams are members of the Morning Glory family (I know, who knew?!) is not even in the same botanical family as the potato. That means Sweet Potatoes do not contain alkaloids. (Alkaloids are substances that *some* people are sensitive to and research suggests they may aggravate arthritis. They are mostly found in the 'nightshade family': eggplants, tomatoes, peppers and white potatoes).

Sweet potatoes are high in fiber and slow to digest which means a slower release of its natural sugars. *Its fiber is classified as a resistant starch, meaning it is not digested into your bloodstream but travels through your digestive system to your colon. There it becomes a prebiotic fiber feeding good little probiotic bugs in your intestines, thus raising the nutrient absorption of your food, including important minerals like calcium and magnesium. These friendly bacteria make many wonderful substances our bodies need, such as short-chain fatty acids and B vitamins.*

Resistant starch has been found to promote weight loss because it's not absorbed into your bloodstream, so it doesn't get turned into fat like other carbohydrates. It also creates Butyrate, the same fatty acid found in butter that research indicates may block the liver's use of carbohydrates for fuel. *This means our body would need to burn fat as an alternative fuel source.* **It also increases satiety producing hormones and staves off hunger because it's bulky and satisfying.**

While research shows that resistant starch improves blood glucose levels and decreases insulin resistance, **in contrast, the starch found in wheat flour digests quickly and is sent directly into our bloodstream.** Once cooked and cooled, resistant starch becomes even more resistant to digestion. And surprise! Our demure, *mild-tasting,* little sweet potatoes can replace white flour, oil, and some of the sweetener in many of these recipes.

I often use the yellow sweet potato and sometimes the orange one; known as the yam, here in America (although we often interchange the names). They're both easily accessible. If you come across any of the various other colors such as purple (I use these to make beautiful Lavender Cupcakes) or the white variety, by all means be brave and experiment. In addition to all their other great benefits, sweet potatoes are also high in antioxidant compounds and are a great source of vitamins and minerals such as C, A, B6, copper, manganese and iron.

NOTE: *If you are eating extremely low carb, please note that the typical recipe calls for 2/3 C of sweet potato, which converts to less than 1 tablespoon per cupcake. You may also substitute the sweet potato with summer squash and a tablespoon of coconut flour if you prefer.*

SUMMER SQUASH

Summer Squash belong to the same family of plants as Winter Squashes, Cucumbers and Melons and are popular all over the world. Scientists have found squash seeds preserved in caves in Mexico and Central America dating back 10,000 years!

Often, people think of the winter varieties when they think of squash, like Pumpkin, Acorn or Butternut. While I use Winter Squash in some recipes, I primarily use Summer varieties for their great versatility and mild flavors. Zucchini and Crookneck, both green and yellow, are two of my favorites because they're full of fiber, vitamins, minerals and other anti-oxidants. Research shows excellent retention of antioxidant activity even after steaming and freezing. Summer Squash even Omega 3 Fatty Acids (in the seeds), and has an unusually high amount of pectin that has been linked with better insulin regulation.

NOTE: *While some of my Frosting Recipes use small amounts of baked Sweet Potatoes (they keep for up to a week in the refrigerator and can also make a quick snack or side dish) the Cupcake Recipes call for Raw Potatoes and fresh or frozen Fruits and Veggies to be pureed into the batter while still raw, making it super quick and convenient!*

OTHER WHOLE FRUITS and VEGGIES

I don't think I have to tout the health benefits of Real Whole Fruits and Veggies in comparison to ingredients such as flour, sugar, bad oils and starches. I think I've made the differences clear already. **These recipes replace those undesirable ingredients with delicious Fruits and Veggies, which for the most part are not even detectable in the recipe.**

The most commonly used Fruits and Vegetables in this book are: Coconut, Zucchini and Yellow Squash, Sweet Potatoes, Red Skinned Potatoes, Pumpkin, Apples, Bananas, Beets and Beet Greens, Baby Spinach, Dark Cherries, Strawberries, Blueberries, Citrus Fruits, Carrots and Avocados.

POTATOES

Unfortunately, potatoes have gotten lumped in with other, less nutrient-dense, starchy carbs and processed foods. Recent studies have revealed about 60 different kinds of phytochemicals and vitamins in the skins and flesh of 100 wild and commercially grown potatoes. They are not the same thing as a KFC Biscuit! While maintaining a lower carbohydrate diet is healthy, I still enjoy an occasional potato!

Red Potatoes contain about five times the level of antioxidants compared to Russet Potatoes. When the boiled potato is cooled, its glycemic score is about 55 compared to a higher score when eating it warm. The starch in the cooled potato becomes more resistant to digestion, and is classified as a 'Resistant Starch'. It's a rich source of Iron, Potassium and vitamins B6 and C, as well as Protein and Fiber. However, Potatoes belong to the 'nightshade family' and contain alkaloids which *some* people may be sensitive to.

NOTE: *While there is less than 1 T Potato per Cupcake, If you're counting carbs, it's important to note that Raw Summer Squash and a Tablespoon of Coconut Flour can easily be substituted in any recipe that calls for a Potato!*

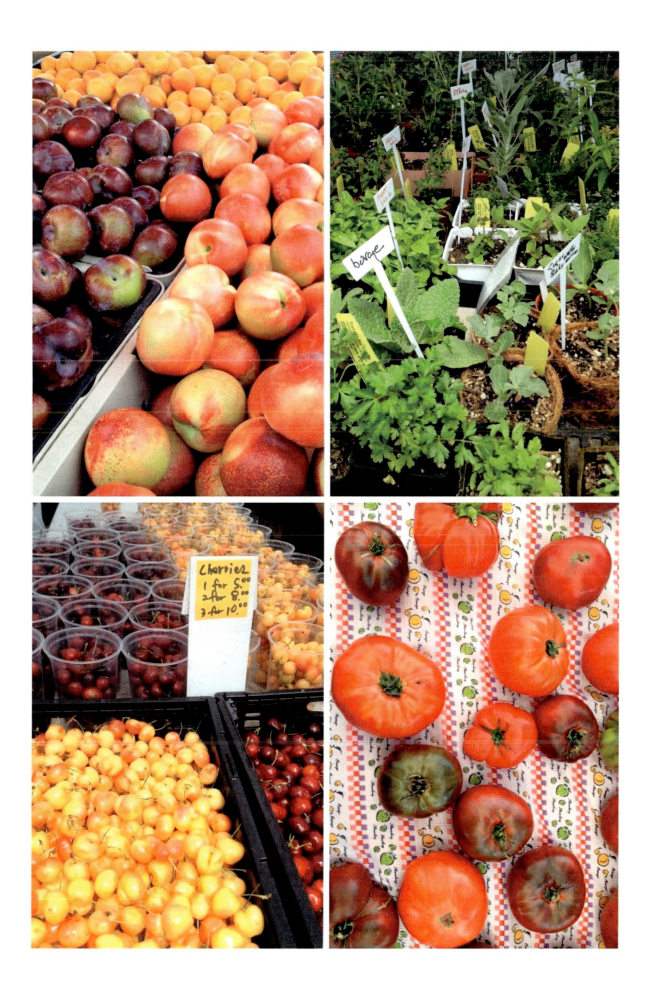

HEAVY CREAM

While you won't find cow or goat milk in any of my recipes, I really enjoy Whipped Heavy Cream on desserts and also use it in my cooking. While coconut and nut milks are other delicious options, in moderation, Heavy Cream has a solid place in my pantry. *Here's why:* First of all, no matter that we can whip up a fluffy topping from coconut cream, in my opinion its taste just can't compare to Heavy Whipped Cream! I also make Sour Cream, Cream Cheese and Butter with Heavy Cream. It provides the fiber to produce Butyrate, a fatty acid that nourishes and balances the pH in the colon, as well as many other functions in the body, one being that it encourages the body to burn fat for fuel (by blocking the liver's use of carbohydrates)! Cream from Grass-fed Cows also supplies us the essential fatty acid, conjugated linoleic acid (CLA), which actually helps keep our cells from storing fat!

I mentioned earlier the big difference between Cream and milk is that *milk contains the highest amount of casein protein.* There is very little casein in Heavy Cream. The lactose sugar is not as big an issue because it should be broken down by good bacteria in the gut (if you're missing it, as many are, a good probiotic supplement should do the job). Most people digest Heavy Cream just fine.

Real (raw, if you can get your hands on it) pasture-fed, Organic Cream is always the best. Pasteurization renders the milk dead and Homogenization denatures its molecular structure.

BUTTER

Butter contains only trace amounts of lactose or casein (clarified butter and ghee contain none) and is usually very easily digested. Butter also makes Butyrate, the same fatty acid we love in both Sweet Potatoes and Heavy Cream. While I use Butter to make some Delicious Frostings, because of the Whole Foods used in these Cupcake Recipes, Butter isn't a necessary ingredient. **I think that just means we'll have to enjoy it more often with other foods, or slathered on my Blueberry, Banana or Apple Cupcakes!** ☺

COCONUT OIL and PALM SHORTENING

Coconut oil is great for baking, but like butter, we don't use much oil because most of these recipes just don't require the addition of it. The Real Whole Foods I use bring with them their own oils. Even good oils are also a partial food and I just think our bodies assimilate and digest the Whole Food better, so Shredded Coconut, with its oil intact, is used in all of these recipes.

As mentioned earlier, Coconut oil is one of nature's rare sources of Lauric Acid, a medium-chain fatty acid which is quickly digested and sent to the liver where it enters your cell's mitochondria and produces energy! This is unlike the long-chain fatty acids found in polyunsaturated oils which your body cannot process as well so prefers to store instead.

Palm Shortening makes great frostings because of its mild flavor, texture and its higher melting point than Coconut Oil. It is simply whipped from Palm Oil and is ***not* a mechanically hydrogenated, fake fat.**

I prefer to use the Whole Foods instead of adding oils to my Cupcakes because anytime we can avoid heating oil I believe it's best to do so. Even with the stable oils like Coconut, Palm and Butter. Heating oil to high temperatures (something often done in processing and that's why you *always* want to buy cold-pressed oils) breaks them down and creates those awful, rogue, free-radicals that run around our bodies, stealing electrons and destroying (and aging) our healthy cells. We've heard a lot about those and how our modern diet creates and promotes the formation of these free radicals. This is just one reason why we need to boost our intake of antioxidants (predominately found in plant foods...and these Real Whole Food Cupcakes!) to counteract this oxidative damage. **Better yet, just avoid the damage in the first place.**

OTHER INGREDIENTS USED IN THESE RECIPES ARE...

COCONUT FLOUR - used in small amounts, Coconut Flour is dehydrated, defatted and ground Coconut. I've found that different flours have varying amounts of fat so depending upon the brand you choose a little more or less may be required.

COCONUT CREAM - substitute for Heavy Cream, if desired.

EGG WHITE POWDER - dried, powdered Egg Whites. (promotes a good rise, but is an optional ingredient-buy pure egg whites with no additives, see Resources) AKA: Egg White Protein Powder.

CREAM CHEESE - it's made with Cream, what can I say?! (used for frostings)

MASCARPONE CHEESE - yep, it's made with Cream! (used for frostings)

CREAM of TARTAR - is a by-product of wine making used as an acidic stabilizer.

BAKING SODA - Sodium Bicarbonate is a safe leavener (rising agent) when combined with acidic ingredients. Its natural mineral name is Nahcolite and is found dissolved in many mineral springs.

BAKING POWDER - a blend of Sodium Bicarbonate, Cream of Tartar and a Starch. The starch keeps this combination of an alkaline and an acid from touching until moisture is added. It then gets a second boost of leavening when the heat from the oven hits it.

GUAR GUM - a soluble fiber, it is a complex carbohydrate derived from the pods of the Guar Tree, native to India. It thickens without heating and inhibits ice crystals when freezing.

ARROWROOT - rarely used in this book, its starch is extracted from various tubers.

SEA SALT - all my recipes call for Sea Salt. Buy the best Sea Salt you can, so it can provide you many trace minerals that our processed white table salt cannot.

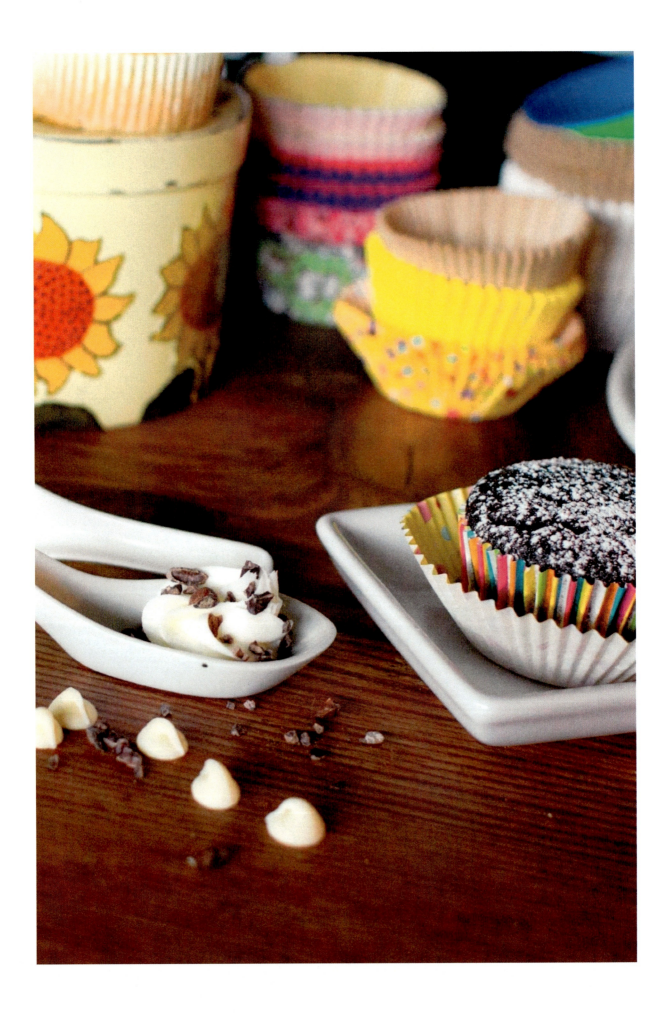

NOTE…Before we move on to Sweeteners… *Pleeease* don't go and make me cry by getting so technical on me that you start pulling the *'that's not really a whole food'* card; because blanched almonds have their skins removed, or that coconut flour has been processed and defatted, or that cream is separated from the milk! Or, that sweeteners…well you know what I'm saying, right? **Let's do the best we can with what we have available to us today and celebrate the fact that these ingredients give us the opportunity to enjoy our desserts and improve our health and waistlines.**

ABOUT SWEETENERS

You've probably figured out by now that I believe our addiction to, and over consumption of sugar, wheat and other refined carbohydrates is severely damaging our health and shortening our life span, so for this reason I also believe some of this information is worth repeating! **WARNING: Sugar is the preferred food for cancer and pathogenic yeasts.** Refined carbohydrates (sugar, white flour, etc.) cause many health issues and combining the sugar with the white flour in your baking just doubles your sugar load. Virtually all the epidemic 'diseases' we deal with today are linked in some way to excess sugar in our bodies.

Our digestive systems use carbohydrates for quick energy by converting them into glucose and glycogen. The body will send this glucose directly to the muscles during exercise; otherwise it remains in the bloodstream, wreaking havoc until being escorted into our cells with the release of insulin. *Because we can't store many carbohydrates, our liver works to convert the extra glucose to fat (which we know we have almost an unlimited ability to store) contributing to fatty liver disease, another growing epidemic. These are just more reasons to drastically cut our sugar and refined carbohydrate intake.*

DOUBLE WARNING: **DO NOT Replace sugar with sucralose (Splenda)!** The nation's number one selling artificial sweetener has had few human studies of safety published. It contains chlorine, has been shown to increase a long-term glucose marker and to shrink the thymus glands, reduce the growth rate and cause fertility problems of laboratory animals.

SWEETENERS USED IN THIS BOOK and WHY

All that being said, in a few recipes you may occasionally want to use evaporated cane juice (less processed sugar) or powdered sugar for a whiter frosting or cupcake, and that is your choice. **I've found that by using erythritol I can easily cut the amount of sugar/palm sugar in a recipe by half without affecting the flavor enough to mention.** UPDATE: Pure monk fruit (drops or powder) is now available and can be used like stevia. The prices of these sweeteners, like their tastes and cooking properties, vary. All of them, unfortunately, are more expensive than table sugar, but for reduced health problems, they're worth every penny.

ERYTHRITOL

Erythritol is my sweetener of choice right now. It's a sugar alcohol that is low on the glycemic index and safe for diabetics. It's classified as an 'unavailable carbohydrate' because **it's not metabolized and is excreted unchanged in urine.** Because these zero calorie carbs are not used as energy by the body, they don't raise your blood sugar, and unlike sugar, **yeast and bacteria in the gut do not feed on it**.

Erythritol is made by breaking down food starch (usually from corn, so buy organic!) into glucose and then fermenting it with Moniliella Polinis (a microorganism found in honeycomb) until it's broken down into this 4-carbon sugar alcohol. Erythritol is also found naturally in many fruits and vegetables, such as asparagus, grapes, melons and fermented foods as well. **Because Erythritol is fermented it does not cause the gassiness that Xylitol or other sugar alcohols can cause**. Xylitol and all other sugar alcohols are made through a hydrogenation process. Xylitol has been clinically proven to fight ear infections and improve the teeth and gums. Erythritol is showing many of those same promising effects.

Erythritol is about 70% as sweet as sugar (however, I prefer to exchange it 1 to 1 for sugar) and is very easy to bake with. An added benefit is that it helps baked goods stay fresh longer. In some cooking applications it may re-crystallize and have a 'crunch' to it (like in frostings). While some enjoy this, to others it may be considered a drawback, but it hasn't kept me from enjoying its other great features.

Use it alone, or combine it with another sweetener. It doesn't have an aftertaste, but has a bit of a 'cool' affect in your mouth. Buy a brand like **NOW Naturals** or **Organic Zero** which dissolve easily. You can also powder it in your blender/coffee grinder for frostings or low-moisture recipes.

COCONUT PALM SUGAR

Coconut Palm Sugar is a lower glycemic sweetener with lower fructose content than table sugar and because it is unrefined it retains its vitamins, minerals and amino acids. The juice of the Coconut Palm Blossom is heated at a low temperature into a thick syrup, air-dried and ground into crystals. Delicious, it has a similar taste to brown sugar (which is nothing more than refined sugar with a bit of molasses added back in). Use it as a 1 to 1 replacement for Cane Sugar.

HONEY and MAPLE SYRUP

Both are sweeter than sugar and contain lots of vitamins, minerals and amino acids. Maple Syrup is made by boiling the sap of the Maple tree and we all know that bees make Honey, which is best purchased in its raw, unprocessed form. While considered 'natural' sweetening options, the obvious drawback is that they raise our blood sugar level because **they are high on the glycemic index scale, so I use them occasionally in moderation.**

DEHYDRATED SUGAR CANE JUICE

This is the juice of the sugar cane, which is dehydrated and generally sold in crystals. It is less processed than table sugar and retains its vitamin and mineral content. **It is high on the glycemic index scale so it should be used very sparingly.** *I occasionally use it in frostings.*

STEVIA-update: PURE MONK FRUIT EXTRACT can be substituted for Stevia

Also known as Rubiana, Stevia is an extremely sweet tasting herb native to South America. It's been used for decades in Japan and other countries but was banned for years from being sold in the United States as a sweetener and could only be sold when labeled as a 'nutritional supplement'. Finally, Stevia is available on our store shelves labeled as a sweetener as it should be. Big companies are now making and promoting products like Truvia, but don't forget what may be hidden in their 'natural ingredients'!

Stevia can have an aftertaste, and is 200-300% sweeter than sugar so it can be hard to bake with. It works well when it's used in combination with another sweetener, such as Erythritol or Palm Sugar. **I also always keep the liquid on hand to add just a few drops whenever I want a little extra sweetness.** *Used sparingly its aftertaste is not noticeable.* You can purchase it at your natural foods store.

PLEASE NOTE: My recipes were tested with the SweetLeaf and NuNaturals Brands of Stevia Powder and Body Ecology's Stevia Drops. I have noticed that different manufacturers can have different strengths and tastes depending upon the ingredients they may use as a 'carrier'. Check your labels and you may need to adjust the recipe amount suggested to suite your brand and taste. (For example one manufacturer I noticed uses lactose as a carrier).

SWEETENER COMPARISONS

	CARBS	GLYCEMIC INDEX
CANE SUGAR	100%	68
COCONUT PALM Crystals/Nectar	92%	35
ERYTHRITOL	0%	1
LUO HAN GUO (Monk fruit)	0%	0
MAPLE SYRUP	84-93%	54
RAW HONEY	82%	35-65
STEVIA	0%	0
XYLITOL	0%	12

*The Glycemic Index is a numerical Index that ranks carbohydrates based on their rate of glycemic response (i.e. their conversion to glucose within the human body)

Read more http://nutritiondata.self.com/topics/glycemic-index#ixzz2ZAPBzdyL

"One of the most important studies in medicine, the Diabetes Prevention Program, found that medication did not work nearly as well as lifestyle changes, and this effect lasted even ten years after the study." -Dr. Mark Hyman, Author of the Blood Sugar Solution

OTHER SWEETENERS

At first, I thought I would only list the sweeteners that I use in this book, and then I decided I'd give you a brief description of other common sweeteners because so many of their labels can be confusing. **I think you will prefer my sweetener choices, but here's some info if you want to experiment further.**

AGAVE

Lower than sugar on the glycemic index, agave 'nectar' is derived from the Agave Cactus and is delicious. However, because it is 90% *processed* fructose it is not in my cupboard.

COCONUT NECTAR

Derived from the blossoms of the Coconut Palm tree, it is boiled down into syrup. Highly nutritious and low glycemic, the nectar is dried to form Coconut Palm Sugar, which I use often.

CONCENTRATED FRUIT JUICES

Concentrated fruit juices, such as a product called 'Fruit Sweet", are boiled down to syrup and are mostly composed of fructose.

DATES/DATE SUGAR

Date sugar is dehydrated and pulverized dates. You won't find them called for in these recipes, but I sometimes use whole, pitted dates in desserts or shakes and date sugar or paste is a quick and easy substitute. With lots of vitamins and minerals and fiber, it has the highest concentration of fruit sugars of any other fruit. While it is high on the glycemic index scale I believe eating in lots of whole fruits!

'JUST LIKE SUGAR' CHICORY SWEETENER

'Just Like Sugar' is a sweetener made from Chicory Root and Orange Peel. Chicory is high in inulin, a dietary fiber that is not metabolized as a carbohydrate and is not digested. Inulin is a pre-biotic in the colon, meaning the good bugs feed on it. Inulin can cause gastric distress in some people, so should be used sparingly. It also contains 'natural ingredients'. For these reasons and its aftertaste I don't use it.

LAKANTO

There are several companies that combine Erythritol and Monk Fruit now, I usually use Lakanto. Easy to bake with, it can be used to replace sugar cup for cup. Buy this at... **bodyecology.com.**

LUO HAN GUO/MONK FRUIT

A vine native to China, Luo Han Guo has been used medicinally and as a sweetener in Japan for decades. Like Stevia, it is much sweeter than sugar but low on the glycemic index. It is now available to be used as you would use Stevia. You can purchase it online through Amazon, Lakanto.com or Bodyecology.com.

MOLASSES

Molasses is a byproduct of refined sugar. It contains the vitamin and mineral content that the refined sugar lost during processing.

SORGHUM MOLASSES or SYRUP

This syrup is made from the sweet sorghum grain which is similar to millet. Its juice is boiled as with Maple Syrup. It's sweeter and lighter in flavor than Molasses.

SUCANAT or TURBINADO SUGAR

Sucanat is actually a brand name for 'sugar cane natural' and, like Evaporated Cane Juice, is a less refined sugar than white table sugar, but raises blood sugar quickly.

SWERVE

Swerve is a combination of Erythritol and Oligosaccharides. (see what I mean? How are we supposed to remember these names?) Oligosaccharides (I have trouble even typing this word!) are derived from fruits and vegetables and are a non-digestible fiber that the good bacteria in your intestines feed on. While it doesn't specify organic, it is non-GMO. My one issue with this sweetener, which is also a cup for cup exchange with sugar, is that it too has a hidden 'natural' ingredient list.

XYLITOL

Derived from corn, this sugar alcohol is similar to Erythritol; however it is made through a hydrogenation process and is not fermented as Erythritol is. It can cause gastric distress so I much prefer using Erythritol.

YACON SYRUP

Similar to Molasses, with half the calories of sugar, this syrup is derived from the South American Yacon root. It's considered a 'prebiotic', as it is high in FOS, or fructo-oligosaccharides (there's that word again!), which feed the good bugs in the belly.

TRUVIA, ZSWEET and OTHER BIG NAME SWEETENERS

While these sweeteners combine Erythritol and Stevia, my two favorites, they hide other ingredients under the label 'natural'. I have grown to not trust these types of manufacturers and prefer to buy organic, non-gmo based whenever possible, and to blend my own for a better taste.

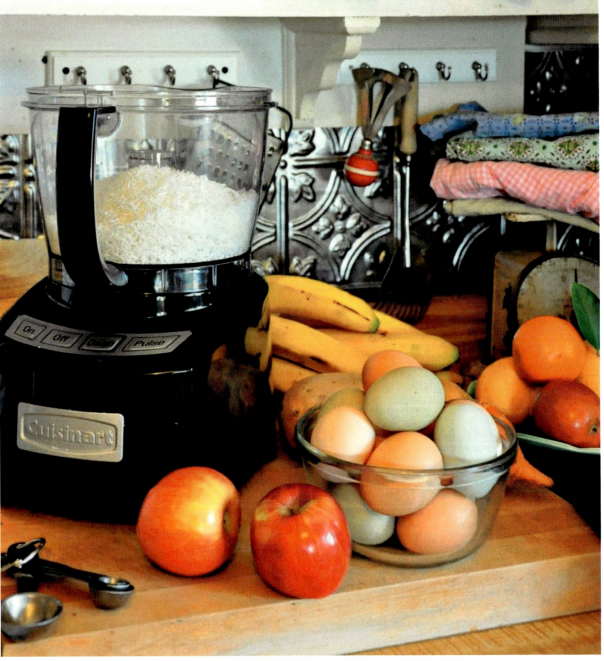

GET READY TO BAKE and BE *SURPRISED!*

REAL WHOLE FOOD BAKING EQUIPMENT

As far as Special Equipment needed, a good Food Processor is it. You can start out with your less expensive model, but will definitely want to invest in a nice, 14 or even 16 Cup, high powered, sturdy model for smooth batter results in minutes. I use the Cuisinart 14 Cup and it's been worth every penny.

I use typical Measuring Cups, Spoons, Spatulas and Baking Pans, nothing too fancy. It's probably smart to get an oven thermometer to make sure your oven is baking at the right temperature. If not, most of us tend to learn our own oven's quirks. I do own a kitchen scale, but rarely use it.

Lastly, you need an oven, which you must own, or you probably wouldn't have bought this book! ☺

HELPFUL TIPS

My passion for experimenting in the kitchen has been a truly enlightening adventure. One of the nicest things about Real Whole Food Baking is that most of the ingredients we use don't require 'add ins' because, it's already there. So, *rarely* do these recipes call for additional oils or liquids… **because the Real Whole Foods already contain them!**

Using these ingredients also brings a short learning curve, because Whole Foods contain different amounts of moisture, oils, fiber, starches and sugars. Once you get used to working with them it's easy to judge whether you need a little more or little less of a particular ingredient. Usually, just adjusting the amount of coconut flour or an additional egg is all that's needed.

While I've always heard how baking is such a 'precise science', I've found that baking with Real Whole Foods can be a rather *inexact* science. *While my measurements may sometimes vary as sizes, shapes and moisture contents of the Whole Foods varies, the final product still comes together and **tastes wonderful!** It doesn't take long to know you may need to leave them in the oven a few minutes longer or add an additional tablespoon of coconut flour to the batter to get the results you want.*

Probably the biggest decision for your ingredient list will be which sweetening option works best for your needs and taste, but **you'll want to wait until you're a little savvier to this type of baking before you make changes to these recipes.** The Cupcakes have the most 'traditional' taste by using Erythritol and Evaporated Cane Juice (sugar), but Stevia or pure Monk Fruit is a healthful option. Sometimes I'll use a little Cane Sugar if I'm making enough to serve a lot of people, because it tastes great and is economical, but still cuts the sugar content in half. **However, as you will see, I usually blend Erythritol, Stevia/Monk Fruit or Palm Sugar to create the sweetness we love without an aftertaste.** I also occasionally use Raw Honey and Maple Syrup. You can do this too by using the chart on the next page for some help on the replacement amounts. Obviously you will get different tastes depending upon the sweeteners you use.

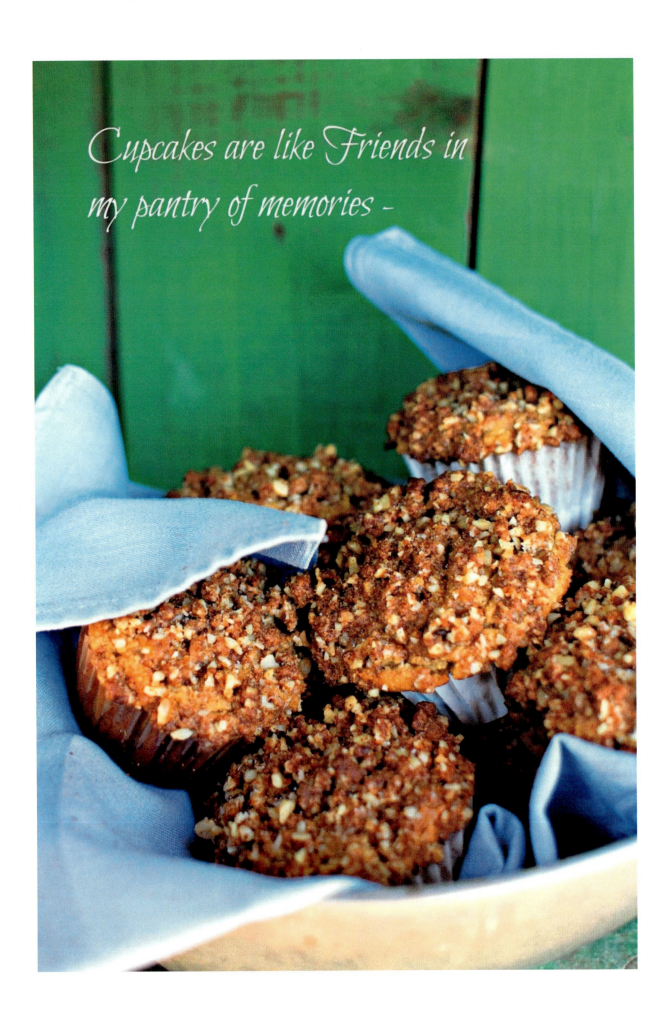

Cupcakes are like Friends in my pantry of memories –

MORE HELPFUL TIPS

1. I once dropped a whole egg, shell and all, into my Food Processor as it was blending, so for this reason I always crack my eggs into a small bowl first, and then add them to the batter.
2. As long as the foods are clean and organic I don't usually bother peeling them (unless I don't want the green zucchini skin to discolor the white cupcake). The potato peel will make a stiffer batter. **Also, taste it to make sure it's not bitter.**
3. Stop your Food Processor and stir and scrape as needed, usually a couple of times is enough.
4. If you don't have cupcake liners, coat the cups with Coconut Oil and dust with Coconut Flour.
5. Once you've added the Coconut Flour and let the batter set a minute, it should be the consistency of thick pancake batter. *Batter consistency will also depend on whether you use the skin or not; the skin will make a thicker, stiffer batter.*
6. **If the batter seems too thick, just add another egg and blend again.**
7. **If the batter seems too thin, add an additional tablespoon of Coconut Flour.**
8. **The Powdered Egg Whites give a nice, fluffy rise, but is optional if you so choose.**
9. Fill each Cupcake Cup nearly full with about 1/3 cup of batter.
10. **If you desire a sweeter Cupcake, I suggest adding a ¼ C of Sugar** (unless you want them to be completely sugar free, of course) **or Erythritol or a few drops more Monk Fruit or Stevia.**
11. When using Erythritol for your frostings, it may re-crystallize and be slightly crunchy; even if it's powdered super fine or melted on the stove. I've found that kids and even a lot of adults like this little crunch! But if it bothers you, you'll have to choose another sweetener option.
12. You may substitute the Blanched, Slivered Almonds for another Nut if you prefer. To de-skin Raw Almonds: Submerge a minute in boiling water, cool and pinch out of their skins.
13. To substitute Almond Flour for Blanched, Slivered Almonds add *after* the Shredded Coconut and Sweetener is blended to a powder. 1 ¼ C Slivered Almonds = 1 ½ C Almond Flour.
14. **If a recipe calls for a Potato/Sweet Potato it is usually used Raw. It can be substituted with a Raw Summer Squash (like a yellow or green Zucchini) or even another fruit/veggie, plus an additional 1-2 tablespoons of Coconut Flour and a tablespoon of Coconut Oil.**
15. **While these recipes use Raw Fruits and Veggies, I also keep Baked Sweet Potatoes on hand in my refrigerator for various uses, like for some Frosting Recipes.** Just place them whole and unpunctured on a cookie sheet and bake them at 325 degrees for about an hour, until soft.
16. I use Unsalted Butter in my Frostings.
17. **To make these recipes friendly for the Paleo Diet Plan, see Tip # 14 above and use the Equivalent Chart for Sweetener Substitutions on the next page.**
18. To make Baking Powder: Combine 1 t Baking Soda, 2 t Cream of Tartar and 1 t Arrowroot.
19. To make Powdered Sugar: Combine 1 C Erythritol, Palm or Cane Sugar and 1½ t Arrowroot.
20. A pinch of Guar Gum added to Frostings increases freezing ability and makes it fluffy.
21. Each 12 Cupcake recipe will also make one 8" Cake round :)
22. Depending upon your oven, these Cupcakes may bake most evenly on the center rack.

CONVERSIONS & EQUIVALENTS

Kitchen Measurement Conversion Tables

Liquid or Volume Measures (approximate)

1 teaspoon	8 pinches/16 dashes	1/3 tablespoon	5 ml
1 tablespoon	1/2 fluid ounce	3 teaspoons	15 ml 15 cc
2 tablespoons	1 fluid ounce	1/8 cup, 6 teaspoons	30 ml, 30 cc
1/4 cup	2 fluid ounces	4 tablespoons	59 ml
1/3 cup	2 2/3 fluid ounces	5 tablespoons & 1 teaspoon	79 ml
1/2 cup	4 fluid ounces	8 tablespoons	118 ml
2/3 cup	5 1/3 fluid ounces	10 tablespoons & 2 teaspoons	158 ml
3/4 cup	6 fluid ounces	12 tablespoons	177 ml
7/8 cup	7 fluid ounces	14 tablespoons	207 ml
1 cup	8 fluid ounces/ 1/2 pint	16 tablespoons	237 ml
2 cups	16 fluid ounces/ 1 pint	32 tablespoons	473 ml
4 cups	32 fluid ounces	1 quart	946 ml
1 pint	16 fluid ounces/ 1 pint	32 tablespoons	473 ml
2 pints	32 fluid ounces	1 quart	946 ml 0.946 liters
8 pints	1 gallon/ 128 fluid ounces	4 quarts	3785 ml 3.78 liters
4 quarts	1 gallon/128 fluid ounces	1 gallon	3785 ml 3.78 liters
1 liter	1.057 quarts		1000 ml
1 gallon	4 quarts	128 fluid ounces	3785 ml 3.78 liters

Dry Or Weight Measurements (approximate)

1 ounce		30 grams (28.35 g)	
2 ounces		55 grams	
3 ounces		85 grams	
4 ounces	1/4 pound	125 grams	
8 ounces	1/2 pound	240 grams	
12 ounces	3/4 pound	375 grams	
16 ounces	1 pound	454 grams	
32 ounces	2 pounds	907 grams	
1/4 pound	4 ounces	125 grams	
1/2 pound	8 ounces	240 grams	
3/4 pound	12 ounces	375 grams	
1 pound	16 ounces	454 grams	
2 pounds	32 ounces	907 grams	
1 kilogram	2.2 pounds/ 35.2 ounces	1000 gram	

Oven Temperature Equivalent

100°F = 38°C   200°F = 95°C
250°F = 120°C   300°F = 150°C
350°F = 180°C   400°F = 205°C

Equivalents to 1 Cup of Table Sugar

*1 1/3 Cup Erythritol
1 Cup Coconut Palm Sugar
1 teaspoon Stevia Powder or Liquid -*varies with manufacturer and product.*
3/4 Cup Honey plus 2 t Coconut Flour
3/4 Cup Maple Syrup plus 2 t Coconut Flour
1 Cup Xylitol
1 Cup Evaporated Cane Juice (powder/crystal)
*I prefer to use Erythritol 1=1 for Sugar

Almond Flour & Coconut Flour substituted for Almonds & Shredded Coconut

1 ¼ C Blanched, Slivered Almonds = 1 ½ C Flour
1- 1½ C Shredded Coconut = approx 3-6 T Flour

'Low Carb' FYI: 2/3 C Sweet/Potato per Recipe = less than 1 Tablespoon per Cupcake!

NOTE: The more fiber, fat and protein in a meal the slower the digestion and absorption of sugars and carbs, therefore a slower blood sugar elevation.

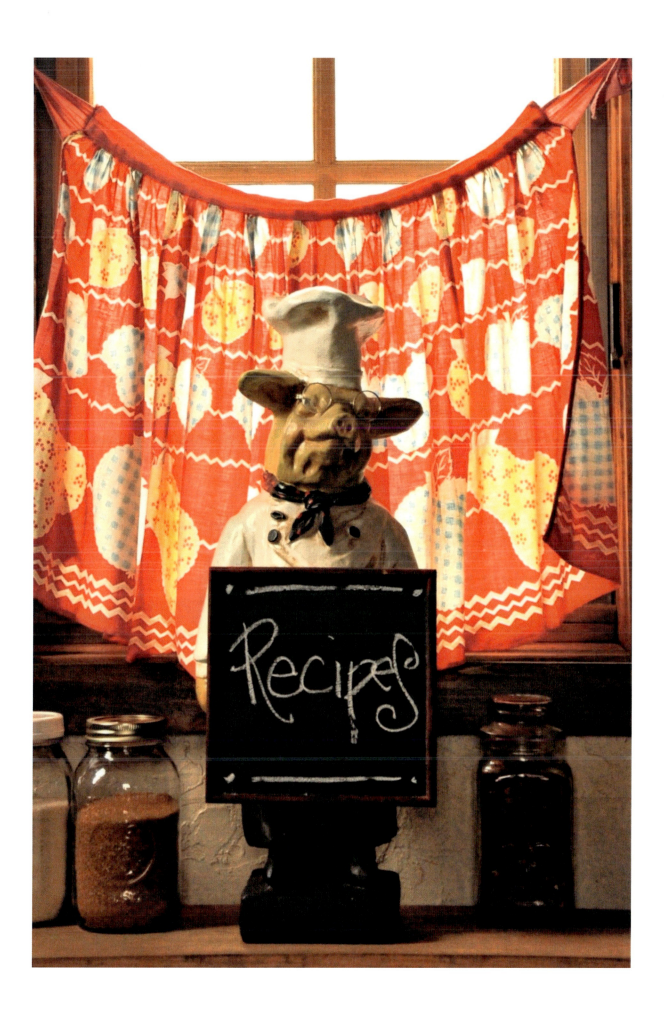

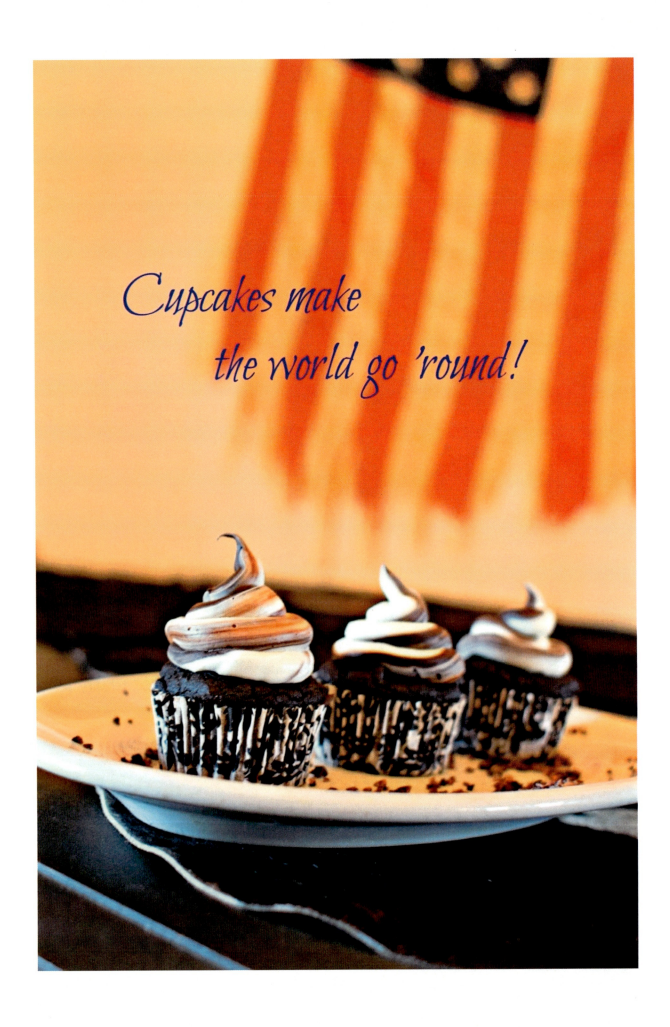

CUPCAKES

Apple Spice	40	Key Lime	72
Banana Nut	42	Lavender	74
Black Forest	44	Lemon Meringue	76
Blueberry Muffin	46	Maple Bacon Bourbon	78
Caramel Cheesecake	48	Old Fashioned Yellow	80
Carrot Cake	50	Orangesicle	82
Chocolate Chip Cookie	52	Peaches 'n Cream	84
Chocolate Soufflé	54	Peanut Butter 'n Jelly	86
Cinnamon Roll	56	Pineapple Upside Down	88
Coconut Cream	58	Pistachio	90
Dark Chocolate	60	Red Velvet Cupcake	92
Devil's Food	62	Rich White	94
German Chocolate	64	S'morelicious	96
Ginger Bread	66	Strawberry Shortcake	98
Green Goddess	68	Tiramisu	100
Harvest	70	Very Vanilla	102

Update: pure Monk Fruit can now be substituted for Stevia.

Apple Spice Cupcakes
Makes 12 Cupcakes

CRUMB TOPPING

1/2 C	Chopped Pecans
1/3 C	Palm Sugar
1 T	Coconut Flour
2 T	Cold Butter
1 t	Cinnamon

Blend together with your fingers, or a pastry blender, into a Crumble. Set aside.

CUPCAKE INGREDIENTS

1 ¼ C	Blanched, Slivered Almonds
1 ¼ C	Unsweetened, Shredded Coconut
1/3 C	Erythritol
1/2 C	Palm Sugar or 1/3 t Stevia
1 C	Chopped Yellow Sweet Potato
3/4-1 C	Chopped Apple (1 medium)
3 LG	Eggs
1 T	Vanilla Extract
1/2 t	Ground Allspice
1/2 t	Sea Salt
1 T	Egg White Powder
2 T	Coconut Flour
2 t	Baking Powder
2/3 C	Peeled and Chopped Apple (to stir in)

DIRECTIONS

Position your oven rack to lower portion of oven. Preheat the oven to 375 degrees.

Line Muffin Pan with 12 Cupcake Paper Liners and set aside.

In your Food Processor fitted with the S Blade, add the Almonds, Coconut Flakes and Sweetener. Process for 2 or 3 minutes until it's powdery.

Add the Sweet Potato, Apple, Vanilla, Allspice and Salt and continue to process until smooth and well blended. Add the Eggs and process into a smooth batter.

Combine the Egg White Powder and Coconut Flour with the Baking Powder and add while the machine is running. Blend for a minute then let the batter set another minute.

Open the lid and check the Batter. It should be the consistency of thick pancake batter. If it is too thin, blend in another Tablespoon of Coconut Flour.

Stir in the Chopped Apple.

Using an Ice Cream Scoop fill the Cupcake Liners about 3/4 full.

*Top this with a Tablespoon of the Crumb Topping.

Bake at 375 degrees for 12 minutes, reduce the temperature to 325 degrees and continue baking until a toothpick inserted comes out clean, about 25 minutes. Cover with Aluminum Foil if they begin to brown.

Cool in pans for 15 minutes, remove to finish cooling on a rack or paper towels to prevent any sogginess.

Cool and serve as is or add decorative dollops of
BROWN BUTTERCREAM FROSTING page 126

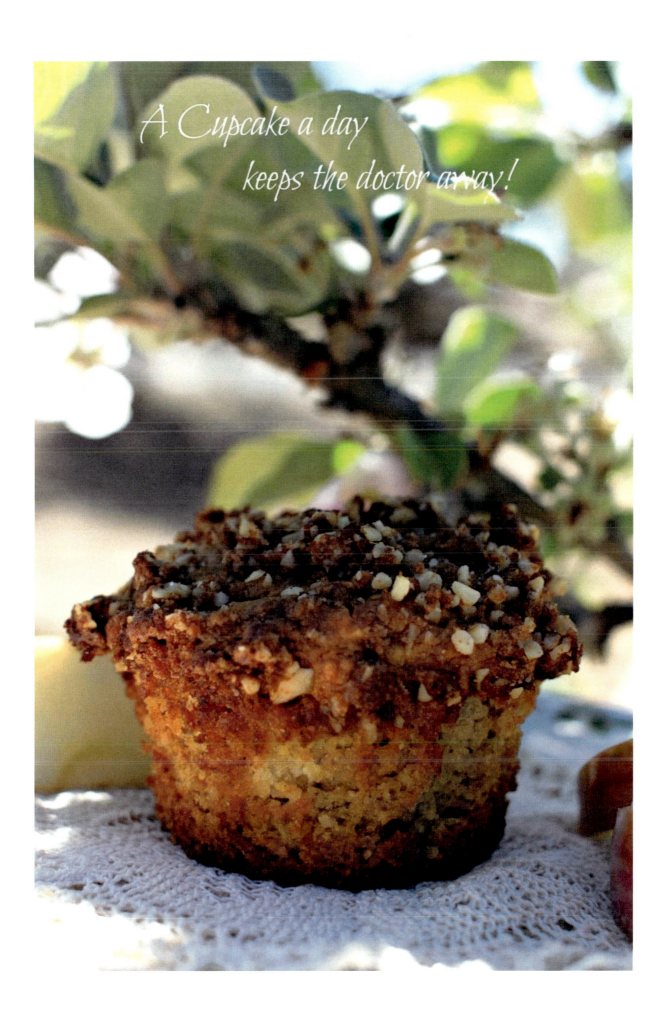

Banana Nut Cupcakes
Makes 12 Cupcakes

INGREDIENTS

1 1/3 C	Blanched/Slivered Almonds
1 1/3 C	Unsweetened, Shredded Coconut
1/3 C	Erythritol
1/3 C	Palm Sugar or 1/4 t Stevia
1 ½ C	Very Ripe Bananas (about 3 Medium)
3 LG	Eggs
1 T	Lemon Juice
2 t	Vanilla Extract
1/2 t	Sea Salt
1 T	Egg White Powder
2-3 T	Coconut Flour
2 t	Baking Powder
1 C	Roughly Chopped Walnuts

*A firm Banana and 2 T Sugar to decorate with

DIRECTIONS

Position your oven rack to lower portion of oven. Preheat the oven to 375 degrees.

Line Muffin Pan with 12 Cupcake Paper Liners and set aside.

In your Food Processor fitted with the S Blade, add the Almonds, Coconut Flakes and Sweetener. Process for 2 or 3 minutes until it is powdery.

Add the Bananas, Eggs, Lemon Juice, Vanilla Extract and Salt and continue to process another minute until smooth and well blended.

Combine the Egg White Powder and Coconut Flour with the Baking Powder and add while the machine is running. Blend for a minute then let the batter set another minute.

Open the lid and check the Batter. It should be the consistency of thick pancake batter. If it is too thin, blend in another Tablespoon of Coconut Flour.

Remove the S blade and stir in the Walnuts.

Using an Ice Cream Scoop, fill the Cupcake Liners about 3/4 full.

Bake at 375 degrees for 12 minutes, reduce the temperature to 325 degrees and continue baking until a toothpick inserted comes out clean, about another 25 minutes. Cover with Aluminum Foil if they begin to brown.

Cool in pans for 15 minutes, remove to finish cooling on a rack or paper towels to prevent any sogginess.

TIP: Use Stevia if you need it to be Sugar Free, otherwise the Palm Sugar adds a nice flavor to this recipe!

Serve as is or frost with a swirl of:
BROWN BUTTERCREAM FROSTING page 126

Top with two slices of firm Banana dipped in Lemon Juice and then dipped in Palm Sugar

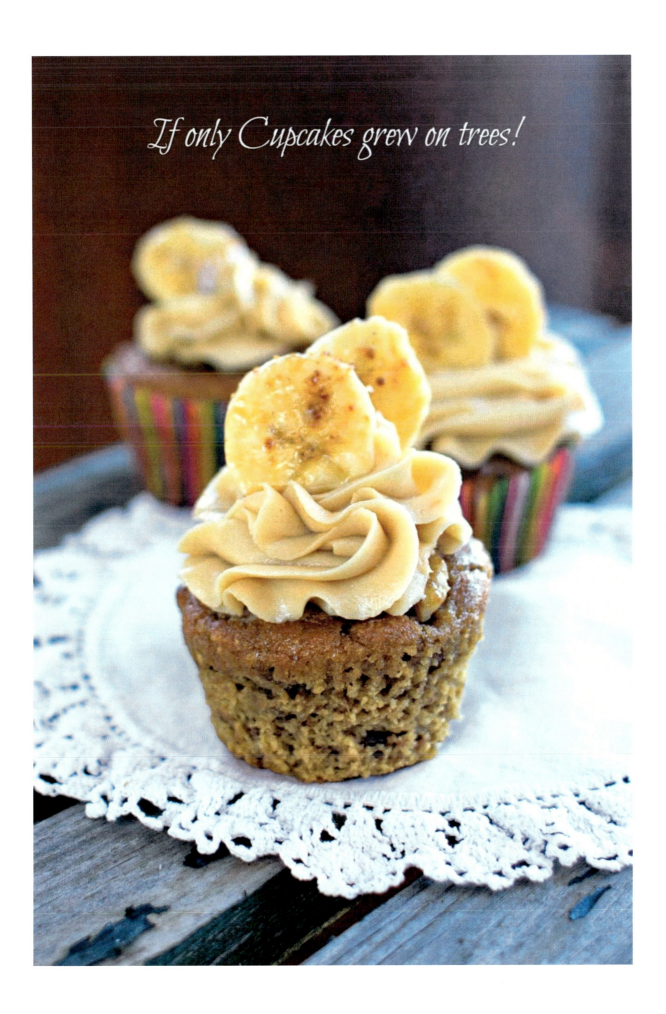

Black Forest Cupcakes

Makes 12 Cupcakes

INGREDIENTS

1 ¼ C	Blanched, Slivered Almonds
1 ¼ C	Unsweetened, Shredded Coconut
1/2 C	Erythritol
1/2 C	Palm Sugar or 1/3 t Stevia
2/3 C	Chopped Yellow Sweet Potato or Yam
1 C	Packed Baby Spinach or Chopped Zucchini
1/2 C	Cocoa Powder
4 LG	Eggs
1 T	Vanilla Extract
1 T	Brandy or Bourbon
1/2 t	Sea Salt
1 T	Egg White Powder
1-2 T	Coconut Flour
2 t	Baking Powder
1 C	Pitted Black Cherries
1/2 C	Chocolate Chips
12	Pitted Black Cherries for garnish

DIRECTIONS

Position your oven rack to lower portion of oven. Preheat the oven to 375 degrees. Line Muffin Pan with 12 Cupcake Paper Liners and set aside.

In your Food Processor fitted with the S Blade, add the Almonds, Coconut Flakes and Sweetener. Process for 2 or 3 minutes until it's powdery.

Add the Sweet Potato, Spinach or Yam, Squash or Zucchini, Cocoa Powder, Vanilla, Salt and Brandy or Bourbon (if using). Process until smooth. Add the Eggs and continue to process into a smooth batter.

Combine the Egg White Powder and Coconut Flour with the Baking Powder and add while the machine is running. Blend for a minute, then let set another minute.

Open the lid and check the Batter. It should be the consistency of thick pancake batter. If it's too thin add another Tablespoon of Coconut Flour and blend again.

Add the Cup of Cherries and pulse a few times to rough chop. Stir in the Chocolate Chips.

Using an Ice Cream Scoop, fill the Cupcake Liners about 3/4 full.

Bake 12 minutes at 375, then turn the temperature down to 325 and continue baking another 25 more minutes, until a toothpick inserted comes out clean.

Cool in pans for 15 minutes, remove to finish cooling on a rack or paper towels to prevent any sogginess.

Frost with: **WHITE CHOCOLATE CREAM** pg. 140 or

SWEET WHIPPED CREAM

1 ½ C	Heavy Whipping Cream
2 T	Erythritol
1 t	Vanilla Extract
	A drop of Stevia if you desire more sweetness!

Whip together with your Hand Held Mixer until fluffy.

Garnish with another Cherry on top and Chocolate Curls or drizzle with Chocolate Sauce!

NOTE: Frosting shown is simply a blend of Vanilla and Chocolate Buttercream in the piping bag!

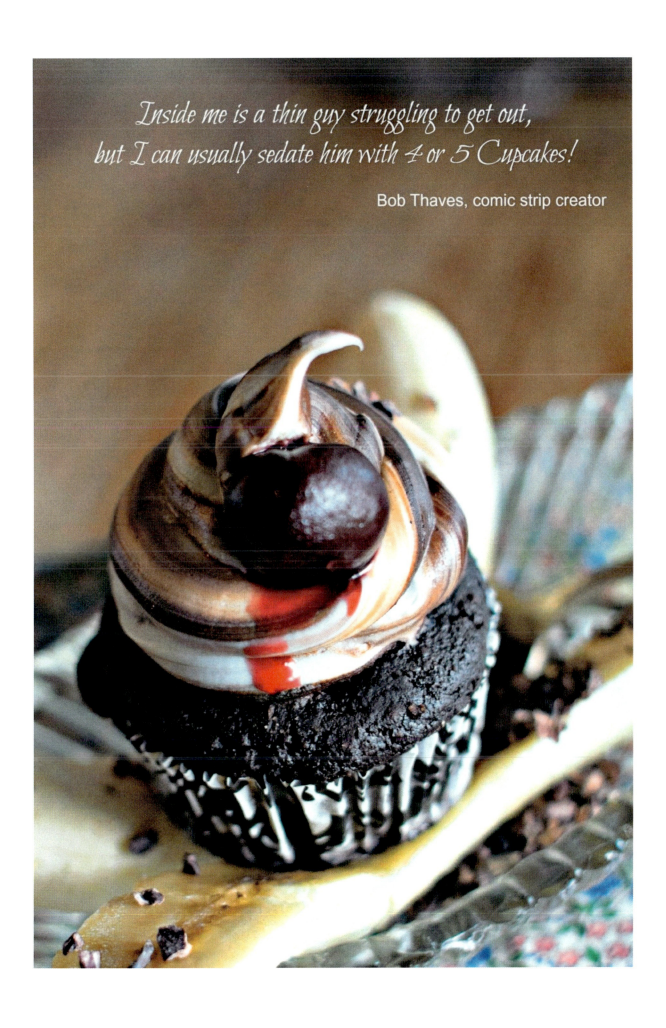

Blueberry Muffin Cupcakes
Makes 12 Cupcakes

INGREDIENTS

1 ¼ C	Blanched, Slivered Almonds
1 ¼ C	Unsweetened, Shredded Coconut
1/3 C	Erythritol
1/3 C	Palm Sugar or 1/4 t Stevia powder
1 C	Chopped, Yellow Sweet Potato
1 ½ C	Yellow Summer Squash or Peeled, chopped Zucchini (about 1 medium)
3 LG	Eggs
1 T	Fresh Lemon Juice
1 T	Vanilla Extract
1 t	Almond Extract
1/2 t	Sea Salt
1 T	Egg White Powder
2 T	Coconut Flour
2 t	Baking Powder
1 C	Fresh or previously Frozen and rinsed Blueberries

DIRECTIONS

Position your oven rack to lower portion of oven. Preheat the oven to 375 degrees. Line Muffin Pan with 12 Cupcake Paper Liners. Set aside.

In your Food Processor fitted with the S Blade, add the Almonds, Coconut and Sweetener. Process for 2 or 3 minutes until it's powdery.

Add the Sweet Potato, Zucchini or Squash, Lemon Juice, Extracts and Salt. Process until smooth.

Add the Eggs and continue to process another minute until smooth and well blended.

Combine the Egg White Powder and Coconut Flour with the Baking Powder and add while the machine is running. Blend for a minute, then let set another minute.

Open the lid and check the Batter. It should be the consistency of thick pancake batter. If it is too thin add another Tablespoon of Coconut Flour and blend again.

Stir in the Blueberries.

Using an Ice Cream Scoop, fill the Cupcake Liners about 3/4 full. Sprinkle tops with Palm Sugar.

Bake about 12 minutes at 375, then turn the temperature down to 325 and continue baking about another 25 more minutes a toothpick inserted comes out clean.

Cool in pans for 15 minutes, remove to finish cooling on a rack or paper towels to prevent any sogginess.

NO FROSTING NEEDED, but Great with BUTTER!

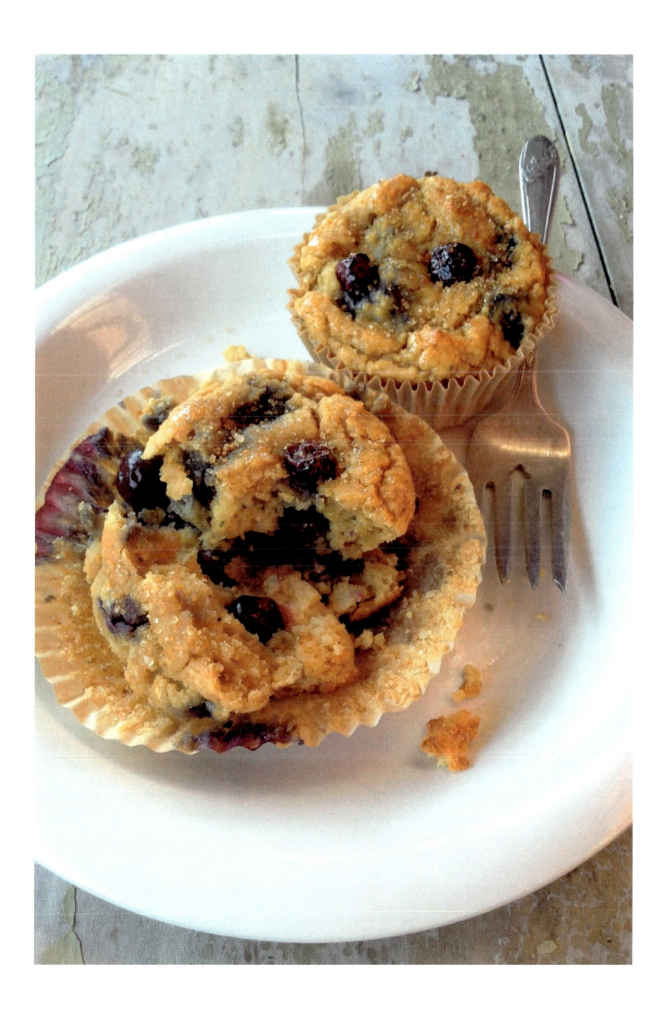

Caramel Cheesecake Cupcakes
Makes 12 Cupcakes

INGREDIENTS

CRUST:

2/3 C	Dried Cupcake Crumbs
1/3 C	Pecans
2 T	Butter

Blend in Food Processor to a Meal. If you don't have Cupcake Crumbs, you can substitute them with another 1/3 C more Pecans and 1 T Coconut Flour.

Press 1 Rounded T into 12 Buttered Cupcake Cups.

CHEESECAKE:

2 C	Cream Cheese
1 C	Chopped Yellow Squash or peeled Zucchini
1/2 C	Erythritol
1/4 C	Evaporated Cane Juice or 1/8 t Stevia
2 LG	Eggs
1 T	Egg White Powder
1 T	Vanilla Extract or Paste
1 T	Lemon Juice
1 t	Almond Extract
1/8 t	Sea Salt

DIRECTIONS

Position your oven rack to middle portion of oven. Preheat the oven to 375 degrees.

In your Food Processor fitted with the S Blade add all of the ingredients and blend until very smooth.

Divide the Batter on top of the Crust. Bake for 12 minutes, then turn the oven down to 325 degrees and bake another 15 minutes.

Remove from the oven and top with the mixture below, *if desired*:

1/2 C	Sour Cream
1/2 C	Mascarpone Cheese
1 T	Maple Syrup
1/2 t	Vanilla

Return to the oven and bake another 5 minutes. Turn off the oven and crack the oven door. Let rest about an hour before refrigerating.

Top with: **DARK COCONUT PALM CARAMEL**

1 ½ C	Coconut Palm Sugar
6 T	Water
2 T	Butter

Combine ingredients in a small saucepan and stir over medium heat until sugar is dissolved. Cover and allow to boil, without stirring, for about 3 minutes, the steam will wash down the sides of the pan. Uncover and boil another few minutes. The Caramel Sauce will thicken as it cools.

If you wish to use a candy thermometer allow it to reach 238 degrees, the softball stage.

TIP: This Cheesecake is delicious alone or with Fresh Fruit also. Peaches and Bananas are especially good if you serve it with the Caramel Sauce!

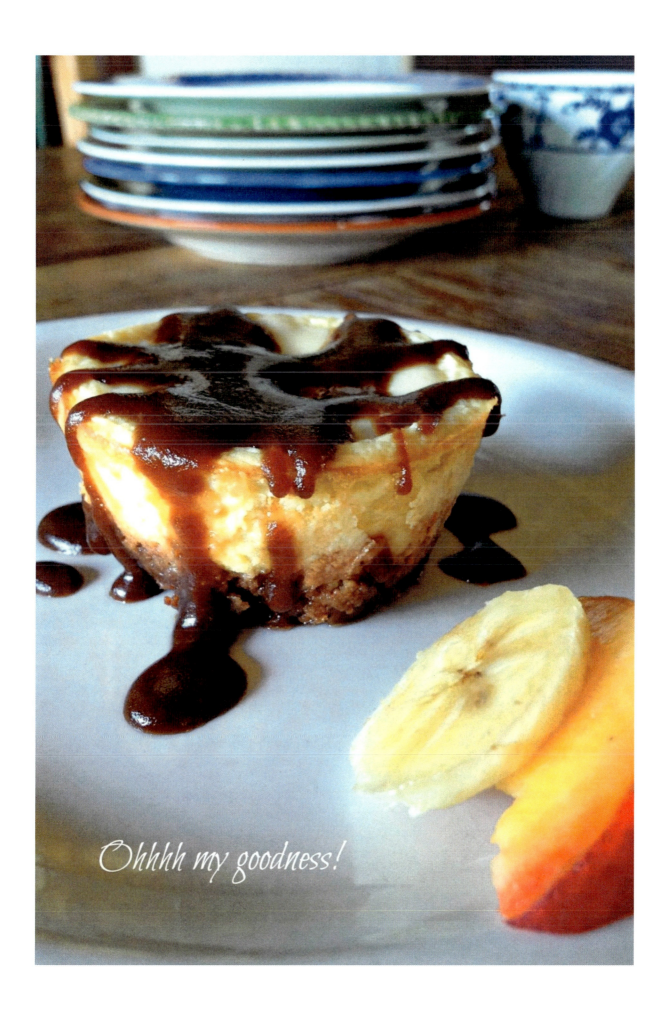

Carrot Cake Cupcakes

Makes 12 Cupcakes

INGREDIENTS

1 1/3 C	Blanched, Slivered Almonds
1 1/3 C	Unsweetened, Shredded Coconut
1/3 C	Erythritol
1/3 C	Coconut Palm Sugar or 1/4 t Stevia
3 LG	Eggs
1 T	Vanilla Extract
1 T	Lemon Juice
1/2 t	Almond Extract
1 ½ T	Cinnamon
1/2 t	Ground Allspice
1/2 t	Sea Salt
1 T	Egg White Powder
2-3 T	Coconut Flour
2 t	Baking Powder

DIRECTIONS

Position your oven rack to lower portion of oven. Preheat the oven to 375 degrees. Line Muffin Pan with 12 Cupcake Paper Liners and set aside.

In your Food Processor fitted with the S Blade, add the Almonds, Coconut Flakes and Sweetener. Process for 2 or 3 minutes until it's powdery.

Add the Eggs, Lemon Juice, Extracts, Cinnamon, Allspice and Salt and continue to process another minute until smooth and well blended.

Combine the Egg White Powder and Coconut Flour with the Baking Powder and add while the machine is running. Blend for a minute then let the batter set another minute.

Open the lid and check the Batter. It should be the consistency of thick pancake batter. If it is too thin, blend in another Tablespoon of Coconut Flour.

Remove the blade and STIR IN:

2/3 C	Peeled, Shredded, Tart Apple (about 1 Med)
1/2 C	Unsweetened Coconut Flakes
1/2 C	Chopped Walnuts
1/2 C	Chopped, dark Raisins or Currants
3/4 C	Shredded Carrots (about 2 Med)

Using an Ice Cream Scoop fill the Cupcake Liners about 3/4 full.

Bake at 375 degrees for 12 minutes, reduce the temperature to 325 degrees and continue baking another 25 minutes, a toothpick inserted comes out clean. Cover with Aluminum Foil if they begin to brown.

Cool in pans for 15 minutes, remove to finish cooling on a rack or paper towels to prevent any sogginess.

FLUFFY CREAM CHEESE FROSTING

1/2 C	Cream Cheese
1/2 C	Powdered Sugar or Erythritol
1 t	Vanilla Extract
1/2 t	Almond Extract
1/2 C	Heavy Cream

In your Food Processor or with your Handheld Mixer, whip the Cream Cheese until smooth.

Add the Sweetener, Extracts and half the Cream and beat 'til smooth. Continue beating while you gradually add the rest of the Cream.

Chill until very cold and beat until fluffy.

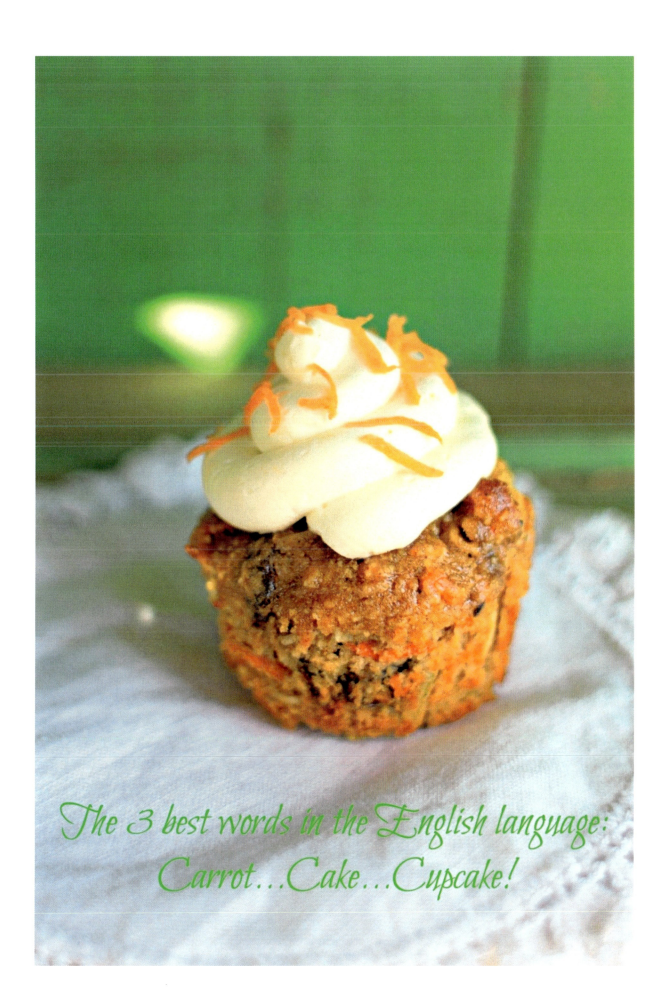

The 3 best words in the English language: Carrot…Cake…Cupcake!

Chocolate Chip Cookie Cupcakes

Makes 12 Cupcakes

INGREDIENTS

1 ¼ C	Blanched, Slivered Almonds
1 ¼ C	Unsweetened, Shredded Coconut
1/2 C	Erythritol
1/2 C	Palm Sugar
1 C	Chopped Sweet Potato
4 LG	Eggs
2 T	Vanilla Extract
1 t	Espresso Powder (not Crystals)
1/2 t	Sea Salt
1 T	Egg White Powder
2-3 T	Coconut Flour
2 t	Baking Powder
1 C	Chocolate Chips
1/2 C	Walnuts (optional)

DIRECTIONS

Position your oven rack to lower portion of oven. Preheat the oven to 375 degrees. Line Muffin Pan with 12 Cupcake Paper Liners. Set aside.

In your Food Processor fitted with the S Blade, add the Almonds, Coconut and Sweetener. Process for 2 or 3 minutes until it's powdery.

Add the Sweet Potatoes, Vanilla, Espresso Powder and Salt and continue to process another minute or two until smooth and well blended. Add the Eggs and process into a smooth batter.

Combine the Egg White Powder with the Coconut Flour and Baking Powder and add while the machine is running. Blend for a minute then let the batter set another minute. Stir in Chocolate Chips and Walnuts

Open the lid and check the Batter. It should be the consistency of very thick pancake batter. If it's too thin blend in another Tablespoon of Coconut Flour and let set a minute.

Using an Ice Cream Scoop or a 1/4 C measure, fill the Cupcake Liners about 3/4 full. If possible, let the batter rest for 5-15 minutes.

Bake at 375 degrees for 12 minutes, reduce the temperature to 325 degrees and continue baking until a toothpick inserted comes out clean, about another 25 minutes.

Cover with Aluminum Foil if they begin to brown.

Cool in pans for 15 minutes, remove to finish cooling on a rack or paper towels to prevent any sogginess.

CHOCOLATE CHIP FROSTING

1 C	Semi-Sweet Chocolate Chips
4 T	Butter

Melt Chocolate Chips with Butter and Stir together well. When it becomes cool enough to spread, frost your Cupcakes!

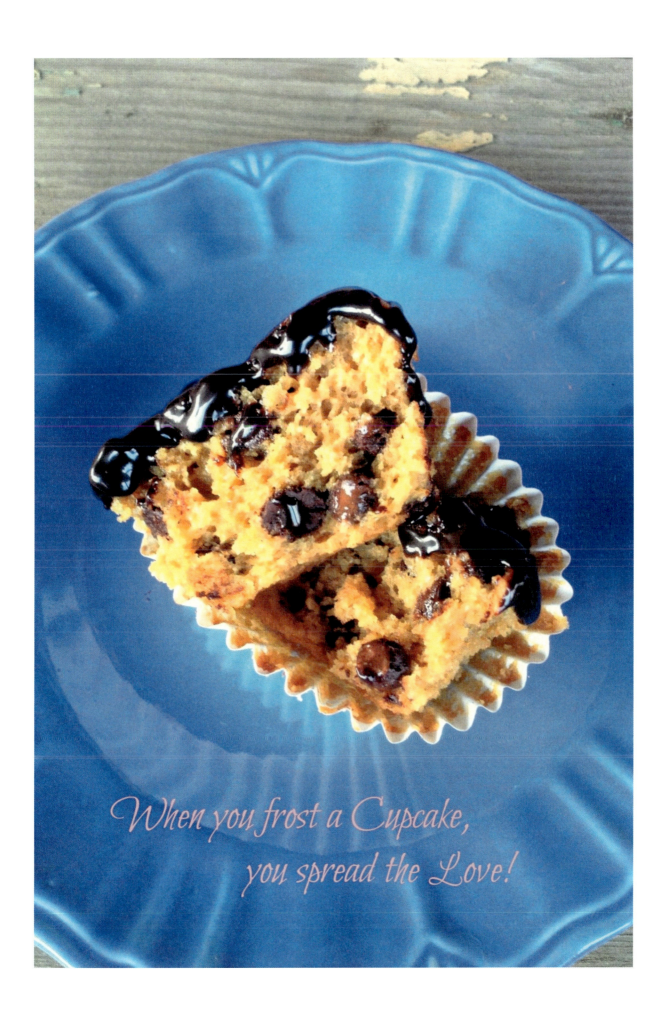

Chocolate Soufflé Cupcakes
Makes 12 Cupcakes

INGREDIENTS

1 C	Heavy Cream
1/2 C	Baked Yellow Sweet Potato
1/2 C	Erythritol
1/3 C	Palm Sugar or 1/4 t Stevia
4	Egg Yolks
1/2 C	Cocoa Powder
2 t	Vanilla Extract
1 t	Almond Extract
1/2 t	Sea Salt
1 T	Coconut Flour
4	Egg Whites

DIRECTIONS

Position your oven rack in the middle portion of oven. Preheat the oven to 350 degrees. Line Muffin Pan with 12 Cupcake Paper Liners and set aside.

In your Food Processor fitted with the S Blade, add all of the ingredients except the Egg Whites. Process this into a nice smooth batter.

In a clean bowl, whip the Egg Whites to stiff peaks but not dry.

Add about 1/3 of the Egg Whites into the Batter and pulse a few times to incorporate and lighten the batter.

Remove the S Blade and gently fold the lightened batter into the Egg Whites until most of the white streaks are gone.

Using an Ice Cream Scoop, fill the Cupcake Liners about 3/4 full.

Bake at 350 for about 16-18 minutes until they're nice and puffy.

Remove from the oven to cool. The Cupcakes will almost immediately begin to sink in the middle. This is *good* and indicative of a Soufflé!

Cool and top with Sweetened Whipped Cream or:

WHITE CHOCOLATE CREAM FROSTING

1/4 C	Chopped White Chocolate
1 C	Heavy Cream
1/2 t	Vanilla

Melt the White Chocolate in the Heavy Cream, add the Vanilla. Chill until very cold and whip to soft peaks.

Add dollops on top of each Cupcake and dust with Cocoa Powder.

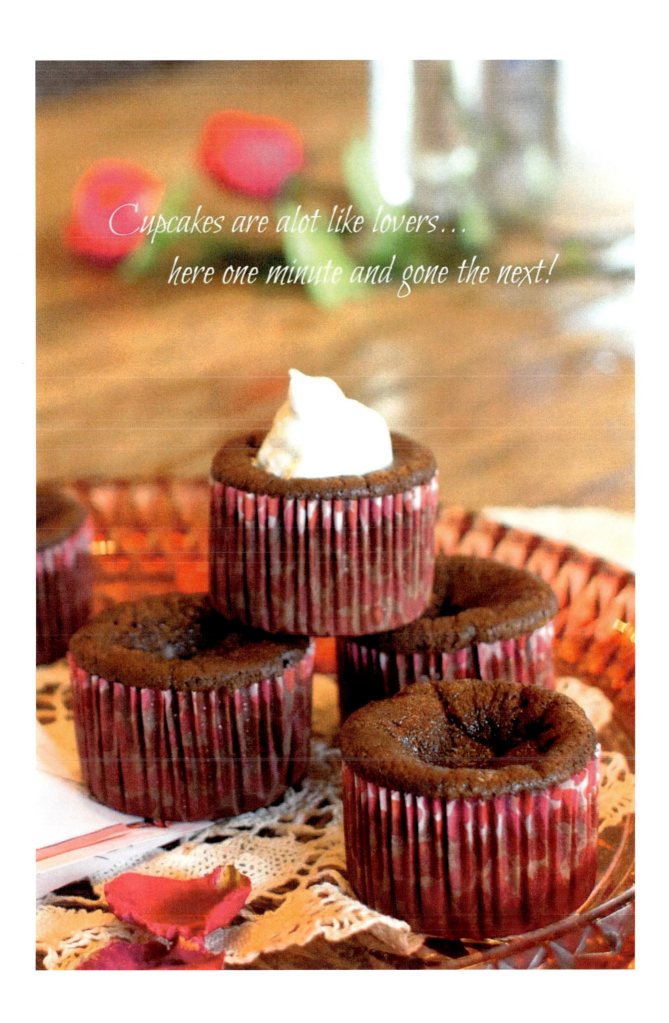

Cinnamon Roll Cupcakes
Makes 12 Cupcakes

FILLING INGREDIENTS

1/3 C	Melted Butter
3 T	Palm Sugar
2 T	Erythritol
1 ½ T	Cinnamon

Mix all the ingredients together and set aside while you make the Cupcakes.

CUPCAKE INGREDIENTS

1 ½ C	Blanched, Slivered Almonds
1 C	Unsweetened, Shredded Coconut
1/2 C	Erythritol
1/2 C	Palm or Cane Sugar or 1/3 t Stevia
1 ½ C	Chopped Sweet or New Potato
4 LG	Eggs
1 T	Vanilla Extract
1 t	Apple Cider Vinegar
1 T	Egg White Powder
2 T	Coconut Flour
2 t	Baking Powder
1/2 t	Sea Salt
1/8 t	Baking Soda

DIRECTIONS

Position your oven rack to lower portion of oven. Preheat the oven to 400 degrees.

Butter Muffin Pan or line with 12 Cupcake Paper Liners and set aside.

In your Food Processor fitted with the S Blade, add the Almonds, Coconut Flakes and Sweetener. Process for 2 or 3 minutes until it's powdery.

Add the Potato, Vanilla and Salt and continue to process until smooth and well blended. Add the Eggs and process into a smooth batter.

Combine the Egg White Powder and Coconut Flour with the Baking Powder and Baking Soda and add while the machine is running. Blend for a minute then let the batter set another minute.

Open the lid and check the Batter. It should be the consistency of thick pancake batter.

Using an Ice Cream Scoop, fill the Cupcake cups about 1/3 full. Top this with a teaspoon of the Filling. Add another scoop of the batter so that the cups are about 3/4 of the way full.

Add another teaspoon of the Filling on top. Use a spoon handle or a wooden skewer to swirl through the batter.

Bake about 8 minutes at 400, then turn the temperature down to 350 and continue baking another 25 minutes, until a toothpick inserted comes out clean.

Cover with Aluminum Foil if they begin to brown too much.

While the Cupcakes are Baking make the Frosting:

BUTTERY CREAM CHEESE FROSTING

1/2 C	Soft Butter
1/2 C	Soft Cream Cheese
1/2 C	Powdered Sugar or Erythritol
1 T	Maple Syrup or Honey
1/8 t	Sea Salt

Blend all the ingredients together and frost the cooled Cupcakes, *or frost them warm for a real Cinnamon Roll look!*

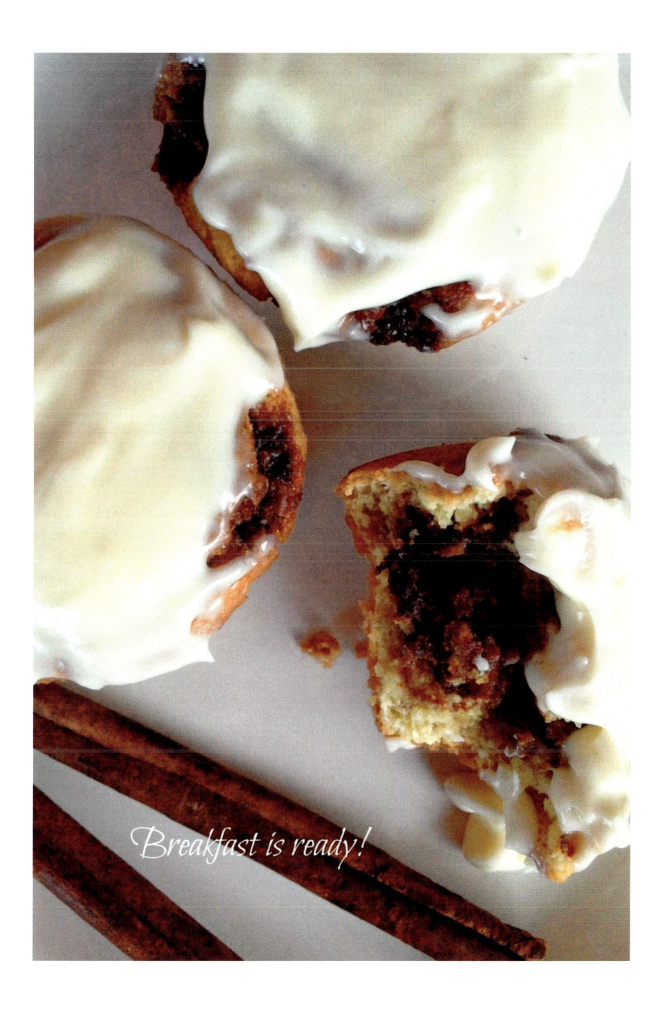

Coconut Cream Cupcakes

Makes 12 Cupcakes

INGREDIENTS

1 ½ C	Unsweetened, Shredded Coconut	
1 C	Blanched, Slivered Almonds	
1/2 C	Erythritol	
1/2 C	Evaporated Cane Juice or 1/3 t Stevia	
1 C	Peeled and Chopped New Potato	
1 ½ C	Peeled and Chopped Zucchini	
2 LG	Eggs plus 2 LG Egg Whites	
	(reserve the 2 Yolks for the Cream Filling)	
3 T	Melted, Virgin Coconut Oil	
2 t	Vanilla Extract	
1 t	Almond Extract	
1 t	Coconut Extract (optional)	
1/2 t	Sea Salt	
1 T	Egg White Powder	
2 T	Coconut Flour	
2 t	Baking Powder	

DIRECTIONS

Position your oven rack to lower portion of oven. Preheat the oven to 375 degrees. Line Muffin Pan with 12 Cupcake Paper Liners and set aside.

In your Food Processor fitted with the S Blade, add the Coconut Flakes, Almonds and Sweetener. Process for 2 or 3 minutes until it's powdery.

Add the Potatoes, Zucchini, Extracts and Salt and continue to process another minute until smooth. Add the Eggs and process into a smooth batter.

Combine the Egg White Powder and Coconut Flour with the Baking Powder. Add this and the Melted Coconut Oil while the machine is running. Blend for a minute then let the batter set another minute.

Open the lid and check the Batter. It should be the consistency of very thick pancake batter. If too thin, add another Tablespoon of Coconut Flour.

Using an Ice Cream Scoop, fill the Cupcake Liners about 3/4 full. If possible, let the batter rest for 5-15 minutes.

Bake at 375 degrees for about 12 minutes, reduce the temperature to 325 degrees and continue baking about another 25 minutes until a toothpick inserted comes out clean. Cover with Aluminum Foil if they begin to brown.

IF YOU ARE USING THE CREAM FILLING... Cool the Cupcakes, and then with a small knife or sharp-tipped spoon take out a small portion of the center of each Cupcake to make room for Filling:

COCONUT CREAM FILLING

2	Egg Yolks
2/3 C	Heavy Cream or Coconut Milk
1/4 C	Honey or Erythritol
1 T	Arrowroot Powder
1 t	Vanilla Extract or Paste
1 t	Coconut Extract or 1 T Virgin Coconut Oil
1/4 C	Unsweetened, Shredded Coconut (optional)

DIRECTIONS

Stir all the ingredients except the Shredded Coconut together in a small saucepan over medium-low heat until it begins to bubble and thicken. Turn off the heat and continue stirring to release some steam. If there are any lumps, push it through a strainer. Stir in the Coconut and continue cooling until ready to fill the Cupcakes.

Frost with: **SWEET WHIPPED CREAM** or **COCONUT WHIPPED CREAM** page 140

Top with **Toasted** or **Sweet Shredded Coconut**

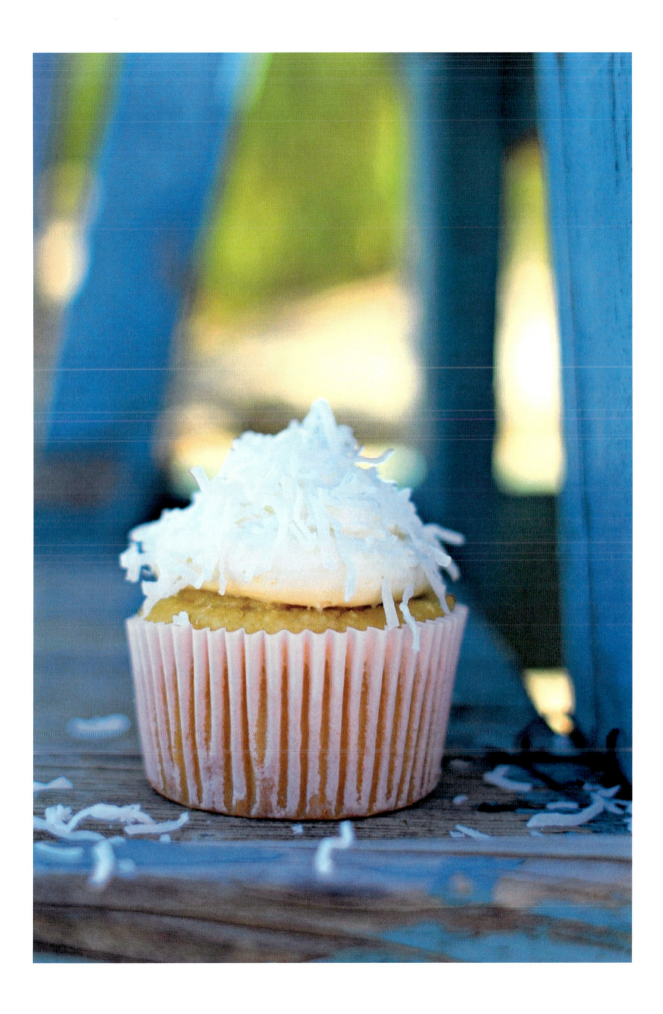

Dark Chocolate Cupcakes

Makes 12 Cupcakes

INGREDIENTS

1 ¼ C	Blanched, Slivered Almonds
1 ¼ C	Unsweetened, Shredded Coconut
1/2 C	Erythritol
1/2 C	Palm Sugar or 1/3 t Stevia
1 C	Chopped Yellow Sweet Potato or Yam
1 ½ C	Packed Baby Spinach or Chopped Zucchini
1/2 C	Cocoa Powder
4 LG	Eggs
1 T	Vanilla Extract
1 t	Almond Extract
1 t	Instant Espresso Powder (optional)
2/3 t	Sea Salt
1-2 T	Coconut Flour
2 t	Baking Powder

DIRECTIONS

Position your oven rack to lower portion of oven. Preheat the oven to 375 degrees. Line Muffin Pan with 12 Cupcake Paper Liners and set aside.

In your Food Processor fitted with the S Blade, add the Almonds, Coconut and Sweetener. Process for 2 or 3 minutes until it is powdery.

Add the Sweet Potato or Yam, Spinach or Squash, Cocoa Powder, Extracts, Salt and Espresso Powder and process until smooth.

Add the Eggs and continue to process another minute until smooth and well blended.

Combine the Coconut Flour with the Baking Powder and add while the machine is running. Blend for a minute, then let set another minute.

Open the lid and check the Batter. It should be the consistency of thick pancake batter. If it's too thin, add another Tablespoon of Coconut Flour and blend again.

Using an Ice Cream Scoop, fill the Cupcake Liners about 3/4 full.

Bake 12 minutes at 375, then turn the temperature down to 325 and continue baking another 25 more minutes, until a toothpick inserted comes out clean.

Frost with: **7 MINUTE MERINGUE** page 141
MAGIC BUTTERCREAM page 136 or

FLUFFY CHOCOLATE FROSTING

1 C	Softened Butter
1/3 C	Chopped Zucchini (optional)
1/3 C	Cocoa Powder (Raw Cacao is best)
1 C	Powdered Sugar or Erythritol
2 t	Vanilla Extract
1/2 t	Almond Extract
1/8 t	Sea Salt
	Pinch of Guar Gun
	Stevia drops to taste

Blend all the ingredients in your food processor until smooth until creamy.

Chill before frosting Cupcakes

TIPS: You may substitute the Butter with Palm Shortening or even a 'just ripe' Avocado!

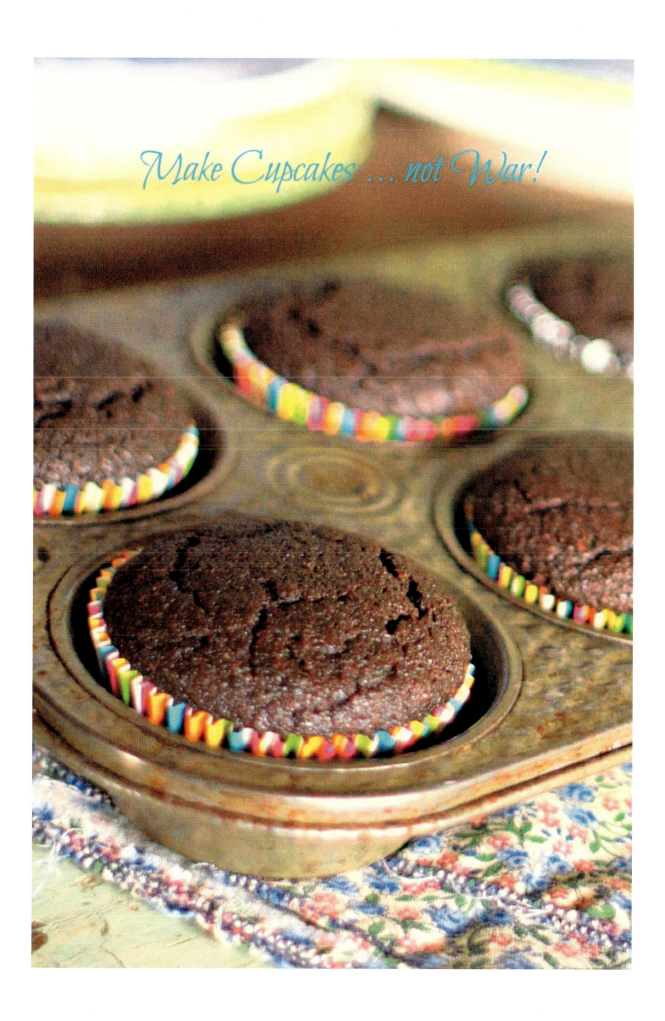

Devil's Food Cupcakes
Makes 12 Cupcakes

INGREDIENTS

1 ¼ C	Blanched, Slivered Almonds
1 ¼ C	Unsweetened, Coconut Flakes
1/2 C	Erythritol
1/2 C	Palm Sugar or 1/3 t Stevia
2/3 C	Chopped Sweet Potato or Yam
2/3 C	Chopped Beet (about 1 Med)
1 C	Packed Beet Greens
1/2 C	Cocoa Powder- preferably Dutch Processed
4 LG	Eggs
1 ½ T	Vanilla Extract
1 ½ t	Almond Extract
1/8 t	Cayenne Pepper (optional)
1/2 t	Sea Salt
1-2 T	Coconut Flour
2 t	Baking Powder

DIRECTIONS

Position your oven rack to lower portion of oven. Preheat the oven to 375 degrees. Line Muffin Pan with 12 Cupcake Paper Liners. Set aside.

In your Food Processor fitted with the S Blade, add the Almonds, Coconut Flakes and Sweetener. Process for 2 or 3 minutes until it's powdery.

Add the Sweet Potato or Yam, Beet, Beet Greens and process until smooth. Stop and scrape sides as needed. Add the Eggs and blend into a smooth batter.

Add the Cocoa Powder, Extracts, Cayenne, and Salt and continue to process another minute until smooth and well blended.

Combine the Coconut Flour with the Baking Powder and add while the machine is running. Blend for a minute, then let set another minute.

Open the lid and check the Batter. It should be the consistency of thick pancake batter. If it is too thin add another Tablespoon of Coconut Flour and blend again.

Using an Ice Cream Scoop, fill the Cupcake Liners about 3/4 full.

Bake about 12 minutes at 375, then turn the temperature down to 325 and continue baking about another 25 minutes, until a toothpick inserted comes out clean, Cover with Aluminum Foil if they begin to brown.

If desired, with your finger, make a hole in the top of the Cupcake and fill with:

CHOCOLATE GANACHE

1/4 C	Semi Sweet Chocolate pieces
1/4 C	Heavy Cream

Melt the Chocolate in the Heavy Cream, stirring until smooth.

Frost with: **DARK CHOCOLATE BUTTERCREAM** page 131 or **MAGIC BUTTERCREAM** page 136

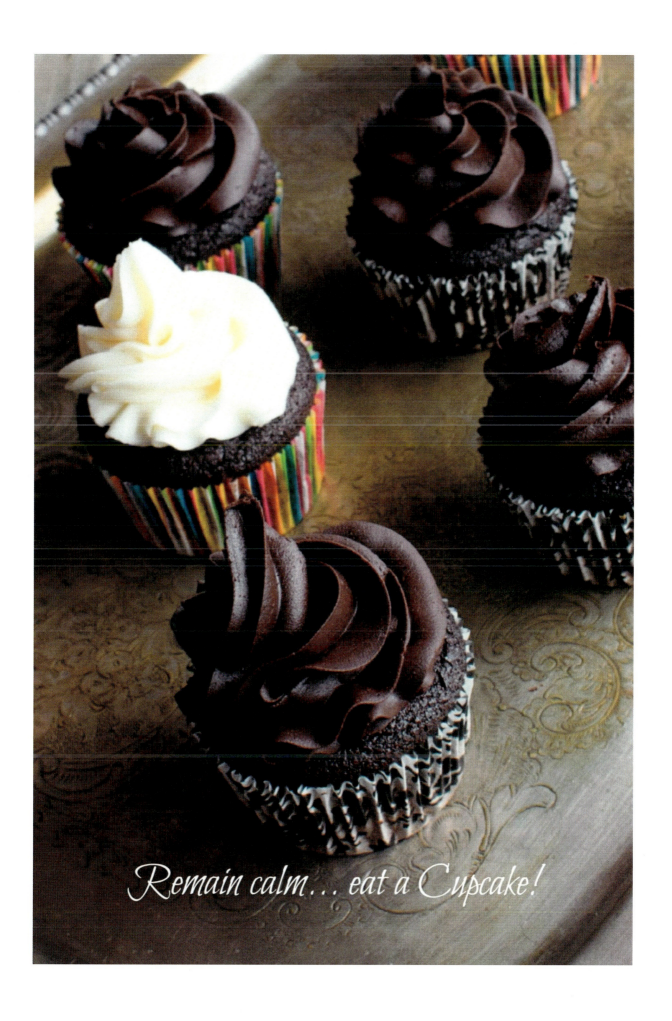

German Chocolate Cupcakes

Makes 12 Cupcakes

INGREDIENTS

1 ¼ C	Blanched, Slivered Almonds
1 ¼ C	Unsweetened, Coconut Flakes
1/3 C	Erythritol
1/2 C	Palm Sugar or 1/3 t Stevia
2/3 C	Chopped Yellow Sweet Potato or Yam
1 C	Packed Baby Spinach or Chopped Zucchini
1 C	Chopped Apple with peel
1/3 C	Cocoa Powder
1 T	Vanilla Extract
1 t	Almond Extract
1/4 t	Sea Salt
2 LG	Eggs and 2 LG Egg Whites *(reserve yolks for Frosting)*
2 T	Coconut Flour
2 t	Baking Powder

DIRECTIONS

Position your oven rack to lower portion of oven. Preheat the oven to 375 degrees. Line Muffin Pan with 12 Cupcake Paper Liners and set aside.

In your Food Processor fitted with the S Blade, add the Almonds, Coconut Flakes and Sweetener. Process for 2 or 3 minutes until it's powdery.

Add the Sweet Potato or Yam, Spinach or Zucchini, Apple, Cocoa Powder, Extracts, Salt and process until smooth.

Add the Eggs and continue to process another minute until smooth and well blended.

Combine the Coconut Flour with the Baking Powder and add while the machine is running. Blend for a minute, then let set another minute.

Open the lid and check the Batter. It should be the consistency of thick pancake batter. If it is too thin, add another Tablespoon of Coconut Flour and blend again.

Using an Ice Cream Scoop, fill the Cupcake Liners about 3/4 full.

Bake about 12 minutes at 375, then turn the temperature down to 325 and continue baking about 25 minutes, until a toothpick inserted comes out clean,. Cover with Aluminum Foil if they begin to brown.

COCONUT PECAN FROSTING

2	Egg Yolks
3/4 C	Heavy Cream or Coconut/Nut Milk
1/3 C	Erythritol
1/2 C	Palm Sugar
1 C	Chopped Pecans
3/4 C	Unsweetened Coconut Flakes
2 T	Coconut Oil
2 T	Honey

Blend Egg Yolks, Cream or Coconut Milk and Sweetener together in a saucepan. Simmer for 5 minutes. Remove from heat and stir in the rest of the ingredients. Cool and frost.

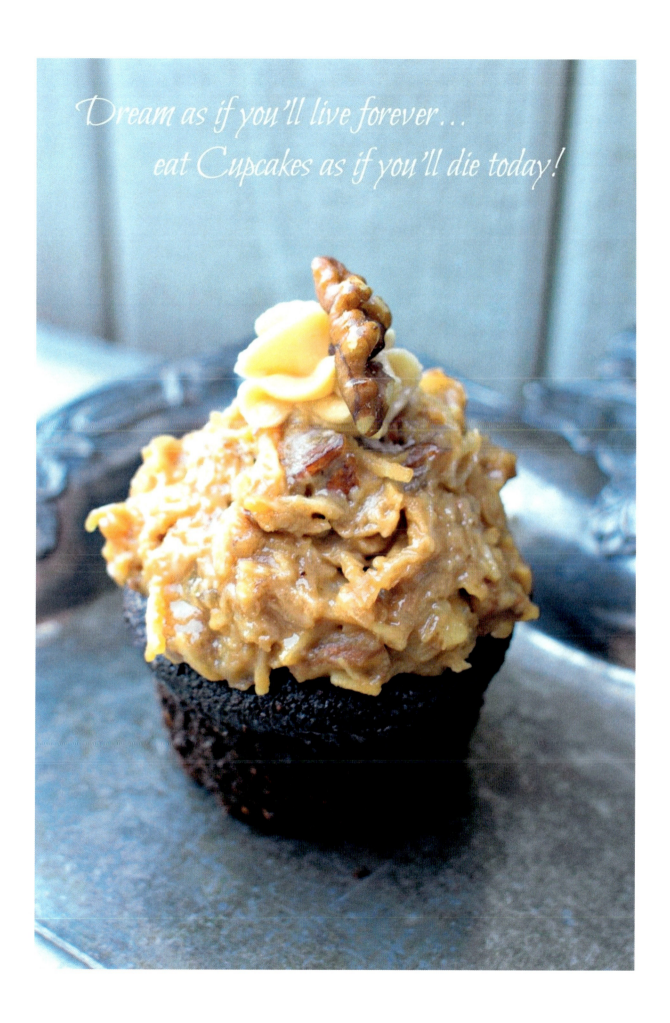

Gingerbread Cupcakes

Makes 12 Cupcakes

INGREDIENTS

1 ¼ C	Blanched, Slivered Almonds
1 ¼ C	Unsweetened, Coconut Flakes
1/2 C	Erythritol
1/2 C	Palm Sugar or 1/3 t Stevia
2/3 C	Chopped Orange Yam or Sweet Potato
1 LG	Orange with Peel, Deseeded and Chopped (about 1 C)
1	2 inch Piece of Fresh Ginger
4 LG	Eggs
2 t	Vanilla Extract
2 t	Ground Ginger
1/2 t	Cinnamon
1/2 t	Sea Salt
1 T	Egg White Powder
2-4 T	Coconut Flour
2 t	Baking Powder

DIRECTIONS

Position your oven rack to lower portion of oven. Preheat the oven to 375 degrees. Line Muffin Pan with 12 Cupcake Paper Liners and set aside.

In your Food Processor fitted with the S Blade, add the Almonds, Coconut Flakes and Sweetener. Process for 2 or 3 minutes until it's powdery.

Add the Yam or Sweet Potato, Orange, Fresh Ginger, Vanilla or Molasses, Ground Ginger, Cinnamon and Salt and process until smooth. Add the Eggs and process into a smooth batter.

Combine the Egg White Powder and Coconut Flour with the Baking Powder and add while it is running. Blend for a minute, then let set another minute.

Open the lid and check the Batter. It should be the consistency of thick pancake batter. If it is too thin, add another Tablespoon of Coconut Flour and blend again.

Using an Ice Cream Scoop, fill the Cupcake Liners about 3/4 full.

Bake 12 minutes at 375, then turn the temperature down to 325 and continue baking about 25 minutes, until a toothpick inserted comes out clean,. Cover with Aluminum Foil if they begin to brown.

Top with: **SWEET WHIPPED CREAM** page 140 or

FLUFFY WHITE FROSTING

1/2 C	Palm Shortening
1/2 C	Powdered Sugar or Erythritol plus 1 T Arrowroot
2 T	Sour Cream
1 t	Vanilla Extract
1/2 t	Almond Extract
1/8 t	Guar Gum
	Pinch of Sea Salt
1/2 C	Heavy Cream
	Stevia drops to taste

With an electric mixer on medium speed, blend all of the ingredients until creamy. Chill until very cold then beat until fluffy. With an electric mixer on medium speed, blend all of the ingredients until creamy. Chill until very cold then beat until fluffy.

NOTE: *Erythritol will re-crystallize and give the frosting a nice 'crunch' that kids love. If you don't want that crunch use all Powdered Sugar.

TIP: To make this frosting Vegan, omit the Sour Cream and replace the Heavy Cream with Heavy Coconut Cream (the heavy coconut cream from the top of the chilled can).

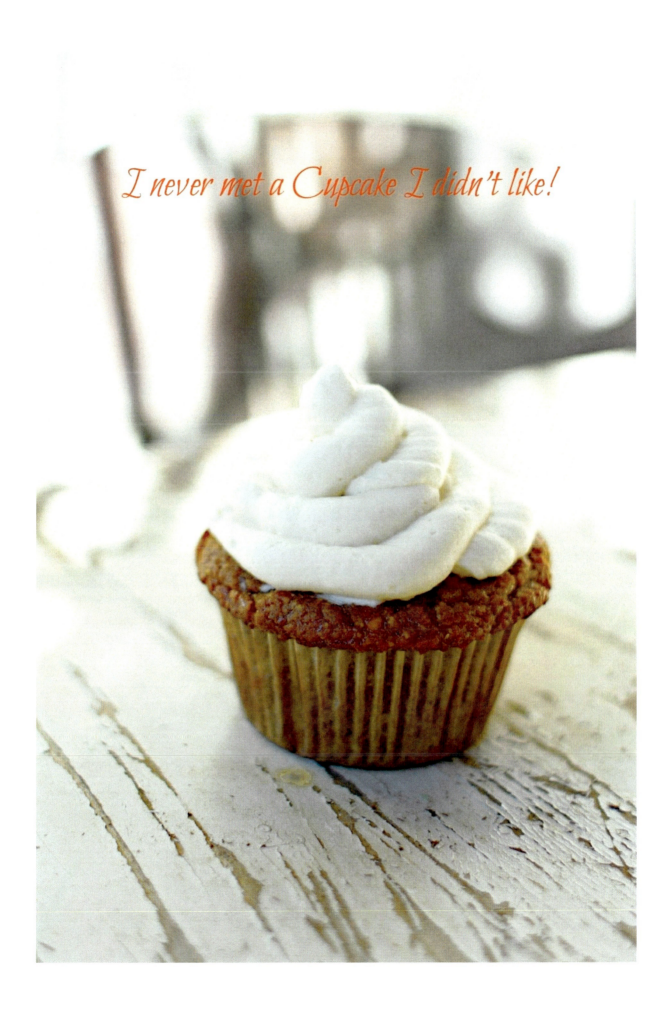

I never met a Cupcake I didn't like!

Green Goddess Cupcakes

Makes 12 Cupcakes

INGREDIENTS

1 ¼ C	Blanched, Slivered Almonds
1 ¼ C	Unsweetened, Coconut Flakes
1/2 C	Erythritol
1/2 C	Evaporated Cane Juice or 1/3 t Stevia
1 C	Chopped Yellow Sweet Potato
2 C	Packed Baby Spinach
3 LG	Eggs
2 t	Lemon Juice
1 t	Lemon Zest
1 t	Vanilla Extract
1 t	Almond Extract
1/2 t	Sea Salt
1 T	Egg White Powder
2 T	Coconut Flour
2 t	Baking Powder

DIRECTIONS

Position your oven rack to lower portion of oven. Preheat the oven to 375 degrees. Line Muffin Pan with 12 Cupcake Paper Liners and set aside.

In your Food Processor fitted with the S Blade, add the Almonds, Coconut Flakes and Sweetener. Process for 2 or 3 minutes until it's powdery.

Add the Sweet Potato, Spinach, Extracts, Lemon Juice and Salt and continue to process another minute until smooth and well blended. Add the Eggs and process into a smooth batter.

Combine the Egg White Powder and Coconut Flour with the Baking Powder and add while the machine is running. Blend for a minute then let the batter set another minute.

Open the lid and check the Batter. It should be the consistency of very thick pancake batter. If too thin, add another tablespoon of Coconut flour and blend again.

Using an Ice Cream Scoop, fill the Cupcake Liners about 3/4 full.

Bake at 375 degrees for 12 minutes, reduce the temperature to 325 degrees and continue baking until a toothpick inserted comes out clean, about 25 minutes. Cover with Aluminum Foil if they begin to brown.

Cool in pans for 15 minutes, remove to finish cooling on a rack or paper towels to prevent any sogginess.

'SPOOKY' AVOCADO CREAM FROSTING

1 Sm	'just ripe' Avocado (about 1/2 C)
1/2 C	Soft Butter
1 Sm	Handful Baby Spinach (about 1/4 C packed)
2/3 C	Powdered Sugar or Erythritol
2 t	Lemon Juice
2 t	Vanilla Extract
1/2 t	Sea Salt
1/8 t	Guar Gum (optional)
	Stevia drops to taste

Blend in your Food Processor until smooth.

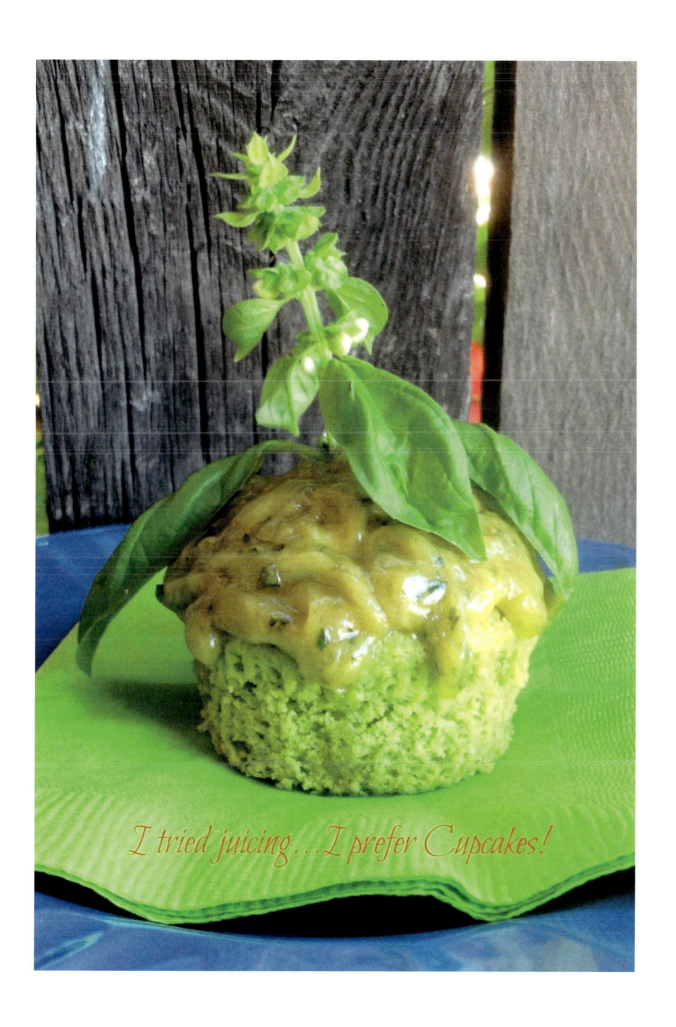

Harvest Cupcakes

Makes 12 Cupcakes

STIR INS:

2/3 C	Chopped Pecans
2/3 C	Rough Chopped Zucchini (about 1 small)
1/2 C	Fresh or Frozen Cranberries
1 T	Palm Sugar
1/2 t	Sea Salt

Pulse these ingredients in your Food Processor 4 or 5 times, until chopped, then set aside.

INGREDIENTS

1 ¼ C	Blanched, Slivered Almonds
1 ¼ C	Unsweetened, Coconut Flakes
1/3 C	Pecans
1/2 C	Erythritol
1/2 C	Palm Sugar or 1/3 t Stevia
1 C	Cooked Pumpkin or Butternut/Acorn Squash
3 LG	Eggs
2 t	Vanilla Extract
1 t	Cinnamon
1/4 t	Nutmeg
1 T	Egg White Powder
2-3 T	Coconut Flour
2 t	Baking Powder

DIRECTIONS

Position your oven rack to lower portion of oven. Preheat the oven to 375 degrees. Line Muffin Pan with 12 Cupcake Paper Liners and set aside.

In your Food Processor fitted with the S Blade, add the Almonds, Coconut Flakes, Pecans and Sweetener. Process for 2 or 3 minutes until it's powdery.

Add the Pumpkin or Squash, Eggs, Vanilla and Spices and continue to process another minute until smooth and well blended.

Combine the Egg White Powder and Coconut Flour with the Baking Powder and add while the machine is running. Blend for a minute then let the batter set another minute.

Open the lid and check the Batter. It should be the consistency of thick pancake batter.

Remove the blade and stir in the Chopped Pecans, Zucchini and Cranberries.

Using an Ice Cream fill the Cupcake Liners about 3/4 full.

Bake at 375 degrees for 12 minutes, reduce the temperature to 325 degrees and continue baking until a toothpick inserted comes out clean, about 25 more minutes. Cover with Aluminum Foil if they begin to brown.

Cool in pans for 15 minutes, remove to finish cooling on a rack or paper towels to prevent sogginess.

Serve as is or Frost with:
BROWN BUTTERCREAM FROSTING page 126

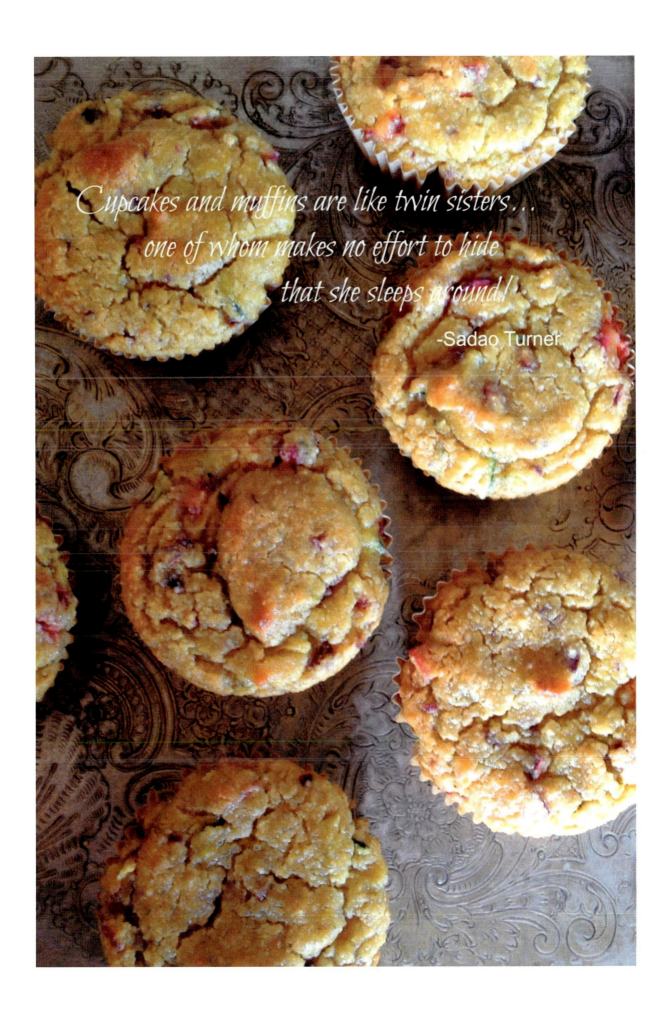

*Cupcakes and muffins are like twin sisters…
one of whom makes no effort to hide
that she sleeps around!*
—Sadao Turner

Key Lime Cupcakes

Makes 12 Cupcakes

INGREDIENTS

1 ¼ C	Blanched, Slivered Almonds
1 ¼ C	Unsweetened, Shredded Coconut
1/2 C	Erythritol
1/2 C	Evaporated Cane Juice or 1/3 t Stevia
1 C	Chopped Yellow Sweet Potato
1 ½ C	Chopped Zucchini
3-4 T	Juice of 1 LG Lime
	Zest of half the Lime *(reserve the other half for the Frosting)*
1 T	Vanilla Extract
3 LG	Eggs
1/2 t	Sea Salt
1 T	Egg White Powder
2-3 T	Coconut Flour
2 t	Baking Powder

DIRECTIONS

Position your oven rack to lower portion of oven. Preheat the oven to 375 degrees. Line Muffin Pan with 12 Cupcake Paper Liners. Set aside.

In your Food Processor fitted with the S Blade, add the Almonds, Coconut and Sweetener. Process for 2 or 3 minutes until it's powdery.

Add the Sweet Potato, Zucchini, Lime Juice, Zest, Vanilla and Salt and process until smooth.

Add the Eggs and continue to process another minute until smooth and well blended.

Combine the Egg White Powder and Coconut Flour with the Baking Powder and add while it is running. Blend for a minute, then let set another minute.

Open the lid and check the Batter. It should be the consistency of thick pancake batter. If it is too thin, add another Tablespoon of Coconut Flour and blend again.

Using an Ice Cream Scoop or a 1/4 C measure, fill the Cupcake Liners about 3/4 full.

Bake for about 12 minutes at 375, then turn the temperature down to 325 and continue baking about 25 more minutes until a toothpick inserted comes out clean. Cover with aluminum foil if the tops begin to brown.

Cool in pans for 15 minutes, remove to finish cooling on a rack or paper towels to prevent sogginess.

COCONUT LIME CREAM CHEESE FROSTING

1/2 C	Softened Cream Cheese
1/3 C	*Coconut Cream or Heavy Cream
2 T	Coconut Oil, melted
1/2 C	Powdered Sugar or Erythritol
1 t	Vanilla Extract
	Zest of the other half of the Lime *(reserve a teaspoon to decorate the tops)*
	Stevia drops to taste

Blend the Cream Cheese with the Vanilla and Lime Juice until smooth. Gradually add the Heavy Cream and whip until fluffy. If necessary, chill in Refrigerator until cold then whip until fluffy.

Frost the cooled Cupcakes and sprinkle with the end of the Lime Zest.

*Cream from the top of the chilled can.

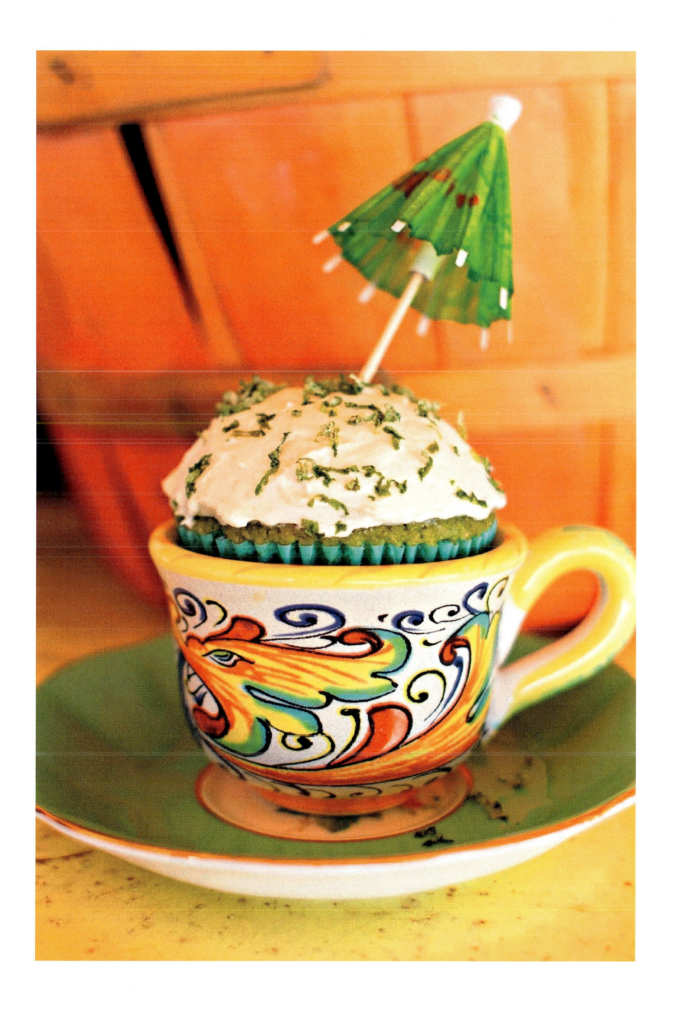

Lavender Cupcakes
Makes 12 Cupcakes

INGREDIENTS

1 ¼ C	Blanched, Slivered Almonds
1 ¼ C	Unsweetened, Shredded Coconut
1/2 C	Erythritol
1/2 C	Evaporated Cane Juice or 1/3 t Stevia
1 C	Chopped Purple Sweet Potato
1 ½ C	Chopped Apple (about 2 medium)
3 LG	Eggs
1 T	Lemon Juice
1 t	Vanilla Extract
1 t	Almond Extract
1/2 t	Sea Salt
1 T	finely minced Lavender Flowers
1 T	Egg White Powder
2 T	Coconut Flour
2 t	Baking Powder

DIRECTIONS

Position your oven rack to lower portion of oven. Preheat the oven to 375 degrees. Line Muffin Pan with 12 Cupcake Paper Liners and set aside.

In your Food Processor fitted with the S Blade, add the Almonds, Coconut and Sweetener. Process for 2 or 3 minutes until it's powdery.

Add the Sweet Potato, Apple, Extracts, Lemon Juice and Salt and continue to process another minute until smooth and well blended. Add the Eggs and process into a smooth batter.

Combine the Egg White Powder and Coconut Flour with the Baking Powder and add while the machine is running. Blend for a minute then let the batter set another minute.

Open the lid and check the Batter. It should be the consistency of very thick pancake batter. If too thin, blend in another Tablespoon of Coconut Flour.

Using an Ice Cream Scoop or a 1/4 C measure, fill the Cupcake Liners about 3/4 full. If possible, let the batter rest for 15 minutes.

Bake at 375 degrees for 12 minutes, reduce the temperature to 325 degrees and continue baking until toothpick inserted comes out clean, another 25 minutes. Cover with Aluminum Foil if they begin to brown.

Cool in pans for 15 minutes, remove to finish cooling on a rack or paper towels to prevent any sogginess.

FLUFFY WHITE FROSTING

1/2 C	Palm Shortening
1/2 C	Powdered Sugar or 1/2 C Erythritol plus 1 T Arrowroot
2 T	Sour Cream
1 t	Vanilla Extract
1/2 t	Almond Extract
1/8 t	Guar Gum
	Pinch of Sea Salt
1/3 C	Heavy Cream
	Stevia drops to taste

With an electric mixer on medium speed, blend all of the ingredients until creamy. Chill until very cold then whip until fluffy.

TIP: You can also use your Food Processor to blend until smooth and transfer to a bowl to chill then whip until fluffy with your Electric Mixer.

TIP: To make this frosting Vegan, omit the Sour Cream and replace the Heavy Cream with Heavy Coconut Cream (the heavy coconut cream from the top of the chilled can).

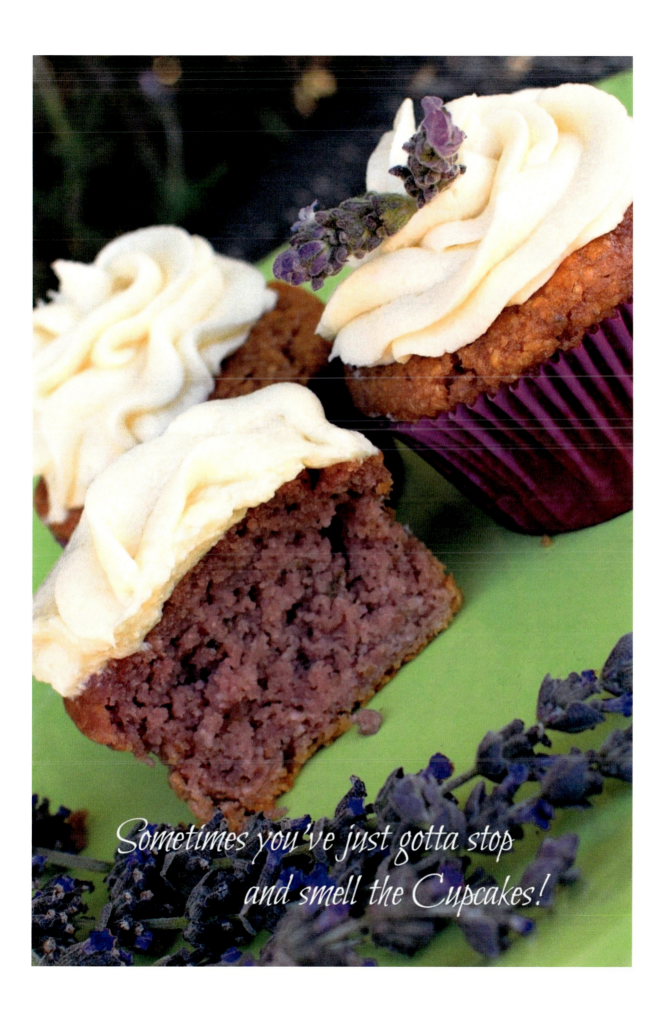

Lemon Meringue Cupcakes
Makes 12 Cupcakes

INGREDIENTS

1 ¼ C	Blanched, Slivered Almonds
1 ¼ C	Unsweetened, Shredded Coconut
1/2 C	Erythritol
1/2 C	Evaporated Cane Juice or 1/3 t Stevia
1 ½ C	*Meyer Lemons with Peel, Deseeded and Chopped (about 2 Med)
1 C	Chopped Yellow Squash or Peeled Zucchini (about 1 Med)
1 T	Vanilla Extract
1/2 t	Sea Salt
1 LG	Egg plus 3 Whites (reserve yolks for Filling)
1 T	Egg White Powder
3-4 T	Coconut Flour
2 t	Baking Powder

DIRECTIONS

Position your oven rack to lower portion of oven. Preheat the oven to 375 degrees. Line Muffin Pan with 12 Cupcake Paper Liners. Set aside.

In your Food Processor fitted with the S Blade, add the Almonds, Coconut and Sweetener. Process for 2 or 3 minutes until it's powdery.

Add the Lemons, Squash or Zucchini, Vanilla and Salt and process until smooth.

Add the Eggs and continue to process another minute until smooth and well blended.

Combine the Egg White Powder and Coconut Flour with the Baking Powder and add while it is running. Blend for a minute, then let set another minute.

Open the lid and check the Batter. It should be the consistency of thick pancake batter. If it is too thin, add another Tablespoon of Coconut Flour and blend.

Using an Ice Cream Scoop or a 1/4 C measure, fill the Cupcake Liners about 3/4 full. If possible, let the batter rest for 15 minutes.

Bake about 12 minutes at 375, then turn the temperature down to 325 and continue baking about 25 more minutes, until a toothpick inserted comes out clean, Cover with Aluminum Foil if they begin to brown.

Cool for 15 minutes, remove to finish cooling on a rack or paper towels.

LEMON CURD FILLING

4 LG	Egg Yolks
1/3 C	Erythritol, Evaporated Cane Sugar or Honey
1 T	Butter
1	Whole Meyer Lemon, deseeded and chopped or just Juice and Zest

Blend all thoroughly in a small Food Processor until smooth, transfer to a sauce pan and cook and stir over medium heat a few minutes until it is thick.

7 MINUTE MERINGUE FROSTING

1 LG	Egg White (use yolk in Filling above)
1/3 C	Erythritol or Evaporated Cane Sugar
2 T	Honey
1 ½ T	Water
1/8 t	Cream of Tartar
1/8 t	Sea Salt
1 t	Vanilla Extract
1/2 t	Almond Extract

Combine all the ingredients except the Extracts in a Double Boiler (or use a Tall Stainless Bowl set on a strainer just above a pan of Boiling Water).

Beat with your Hand Held Mixer for 6 minutes, it will become light and creamy and triple in size. Remove the bowl from the heat, add the Extracts and continue to beat another minute.

I use Meyer Lemons in this recipe. If your Lemons are very tart/have a thick pith, you may opt to juice and zest them rather than using the whole fruit.

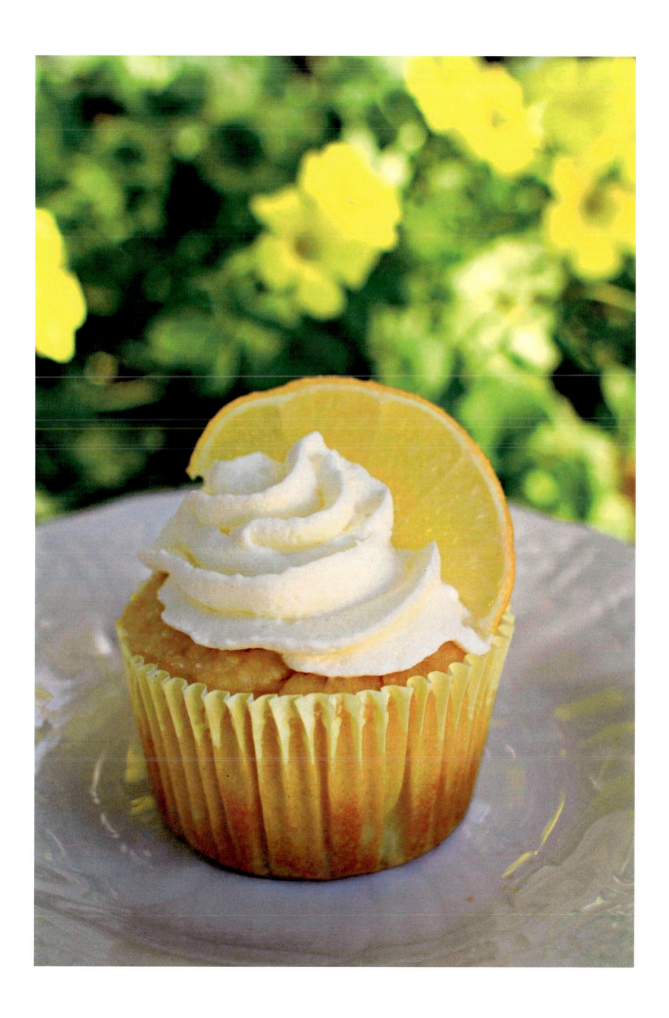

Maple Bacon Bourbon Cupcakes

Makes 12 Cupcakes

INGREDIENTS

1 ¼ C	Blanched, Slivered Almonds
1 ¼ C	Shredded, Unsweetened Coconut
1/2 C	Erythritol
1/3 C	Maple Syrup
1 C	Chopped New Potato or Sweet Potato
2/3 C	Chopped Yellow Squash or Peeled Zucchini
4 LG	Eggs
1 t	Vanilla Extract
1/2 t	Sea Salt
1 T	Egg White Powder
2-3 T	Coconut Flour
2 t	Baking Powder

DIRECTIONS

Position your oven rack to lower portion of oven. Preheat the oven to 375 degrees. Line Muffin Pan with 12 Cupcake Paper Liners. Set aside.

In your Food Processor fitted with the S Blade, add the Almonds, Coconut and Sweetener. Process for 2 or 3 minutes until it's powdery.

Add the Potato, Squash or Zucchini, Vanilla, and Salt and continue to process another minute or two until smooth and well blended. Add the Eggs and process into a smooth batter.

Combine the Egg White Powder and Coconut Flour with the Baking Powder and add while the machine is running. Blend for a minute then let the batter set another minute.

Open the lid and check the Batter. It should be the consistency of very thick pancake batter.

Using an Ice Cream Scoop or a 1/4 C measure, fill the Cupcake Liners about 3/4 full.

Bake at 375 degrees for 12 minutes, reduce the temperature to 325 degrees and continue baking until a toothpick inserted comes out clean, about another 25 minutes.

Cover with Aluminum Foil if they begin to brown.

Cool in pans for 15 minutes, remove to finish cooling on a rack or paper towels to prevent any sogginess.

While the Cupcakes are Baking, make the Glaze and the Frosting:

MAPLE BOURBON GLAZE

12	Slices of Bacon, preferably uncured
1/4 C	Maple Syrup
1 T	Bourbon Whiskey

Fry the Bacon until crispy and drain on paper towels. Crumble when cool and set aside. Stir together the Maple Syrup and Bourbon then add the Crumbled Bacon.

MAPLE/BOURBON FROSTING

1/2 C	Softened Cream Cheese
1/3 C	Soft Butter
1/3 C	Maple Syrup
4 T	Bacon Drippings
1 T	Bourbon Whiskey (optional)

Whip the rest of the ingredients together until somewhat fluffy. Chill until cool enough to spread.

TO ASSEMBLE:

Cut Cupcakes in half and spread with half of the Frosting and top with half the Crumbled Bacon Glaze. Put the top of the Cupcake on and spread with the rest of the Frosting and top with the rest of the Crumbled Bacon Glaze.

TIP: For a 'pancake-looking' top (as shown in photo) fill the Cupcake Cups almost full with Batter.

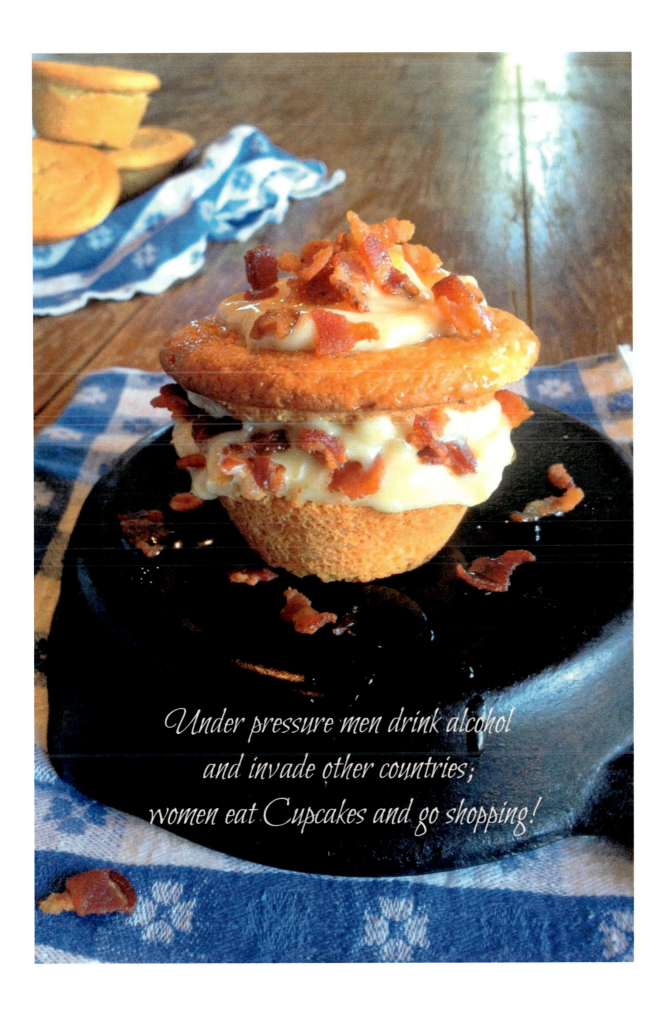

Old Fashioned Yellow Cupcakes
Makes 12 Cupcakes

INGREDIENTS

1 ½ C	Blanched, Slivered Almonds
1 C	Shredded, Unsweetened Coconut
1/2 C	Erythritol
1/2 C	Palm or Cane Sugar or 1/3 t Stevia
1 C	Chopped Sweet Potato
1 ½ C	Chopped Tart Apple (about 2 Med)
3 LG	Eggs
1 T	Vanilla Extract
1 T	Lemon Juice
1/2 t	Sea Salt
1 T	Egg White Powder
2-3 T	Coconut Flour
2 t	Baking Powder

DIRECTIONS

Position your oven rack to lower portion of oven. Preheat the oven to 375 degrees. Line Muffin Pan with 12 Cupcake Paper Liners and set aside.

In your Food Processor fitted with the S Blade, add the Almonds, Coconut and Sweetener. Process for 2 or 3 minutes until it's powdery.

Add the Sweet Potato, Apple, Vanilla and Salt and continue to process until smooth. Add the Eggs and process into a smooth batter.

Combine the Egg White Powder and Coconut Flour with the Baking Powder and add while the machine is running. Blend for a minute then let the batter set another minute.

Open the lid and check the Batter. It should be the consistency of thick pancake batter.

Using an Ice Cream Scoop, fill the Cupcake Liners about 3/4 full.

Bake at 375 degrees for 12 minutes, reduce the temperature to 325 degrees and continue baking until a toothpick inserted comes out clean, about another 25 minutes. Cover with Aluminum Foil if they begin to brown.

Cool in pans for 15 minutes, remove to finish cooling on a rack or paper towels to prevent any sogginess.

MILK CHOCOLATE FROSTING

1/2 C	Palm Shortening
2 T	Baked Sweet Potato or 1 T Arrowroot
2 T	Cocoa Powder (Raw Cacao is best)
1/3 C	Maple Syrup
3 T	Erythritol or Palm Sugar
1 t	Vanilla Extract
	Pinch of Sea Salt
	Pinch of Guar Gum (optional)
1/2 C	Heavy Cream or Heavy Coconut Cream (from the top of the chilled can)

Blend the Shortening, Sweet Potato and Cocoa Powder in your Food Processor 'til creamy. Add the rest of the ingredients, *except* the Heavy Cream, and blend until very smooth. Add the Heavy Cream slowly and whip 'til fluffy. Chill and rewhip if necessary.

TIP: *For a Sugar-Free Frosting with a nice 'crunch' use Erythritol!

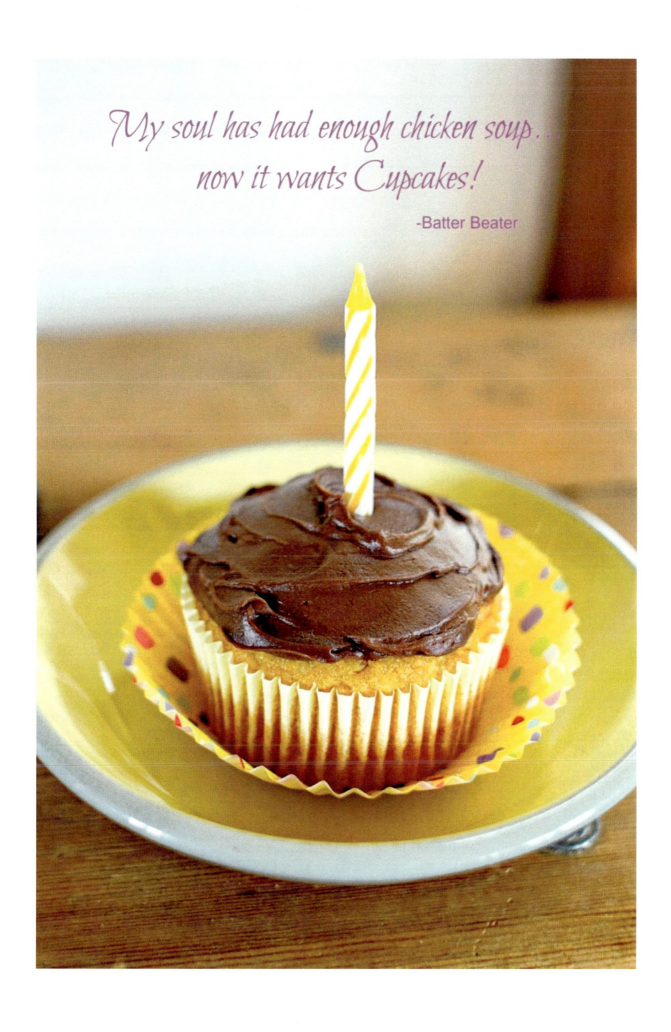

Orangesicle Cupcakes
Makes 12 Cupcakes

INGREDIENTS

1 C	Blanched, Slivered Almonds
1 C	Unsweetened, Shredded Coconut
1/2 C	Erythritol
1/2 C	Palm Sugar or 1/3 t Stevia
2/3 C	Chopped Sweet Potato or Orange Yam
1 ½ C	Orange with Peel, Deseeded and Chopped (about 2 Med)
1 C	Chopped Carrot (about 1 Med/LG)
1 T	Vanilla Extract
1/2 t	Almond Extract
1/2 t	Sea Salt
3 LG	Eggs
1 T	Egg White Powder
3 T	Coconut Flour
2 t	Baking Powder

DIRECTIONS

Position your oven rack to lower portion of oven. Preheat the oven to 375 degrees. Line Muffin Pan with 12 Cupcake Paper Liners and set aside.

In your Food Processor fitted with the S Blade, add the Almonds, Coconut and Sweetener. Process for 2 or 3 minutes until it's powdery.

Add the Sweet Potato or Yam, Oranges, Carrot, Extracts and Salt and process until smooth.

Add the Eggs and continue to process another minute until smooth and well blended.

Combine the Egg White Powder and Coconut Flour with the Baking Powder and add while it is running. Blend for a minute, then let set another minute.

Open the lid and check the Batter. It should be the consistency of thick pancake batter. If it is too thin, add another Tablespoon of Coconut Flour and blend again.

Using an Ice Cream Scoop or a 1/4 C measure, fill the Cupcake Liners about 3/4 full. If possible, let the batter rest for 5-15 minutes.

Bake about 12 minutes at 375, then turn the temperature down to 325 and continue baking about another 25minutes, until a toothpick inserted comes out clean. Cover with Aluminum Foil if they begin to brown.

Cool in pans for 15 minutes, remove to finish cooling on a rack or paper towels to prevent any sogginess.

ORANGE CREAM FROSTING

1/4 C	Palm Shortening
1/4 C	Cooked Orange Yam, skinned
1 Med	Orange, with Skin, Deseeded
1/3 C	Erythritol or Powdered Sugar
1 t	Vanilla Extract
1/2 t	Almond Extract
	Pinch of Sea Salt
	Stevia drops to taste

Combine all the ingredients in your 4 C Food Processor and blend until smooth.

TIP: Use a sweet, thinner skinned Orange.

TIP: The orange Yam or yellow Sweet Potato works equally as well. Simply set on a cookie sheet and bake at 325 for an hour or more until soft.

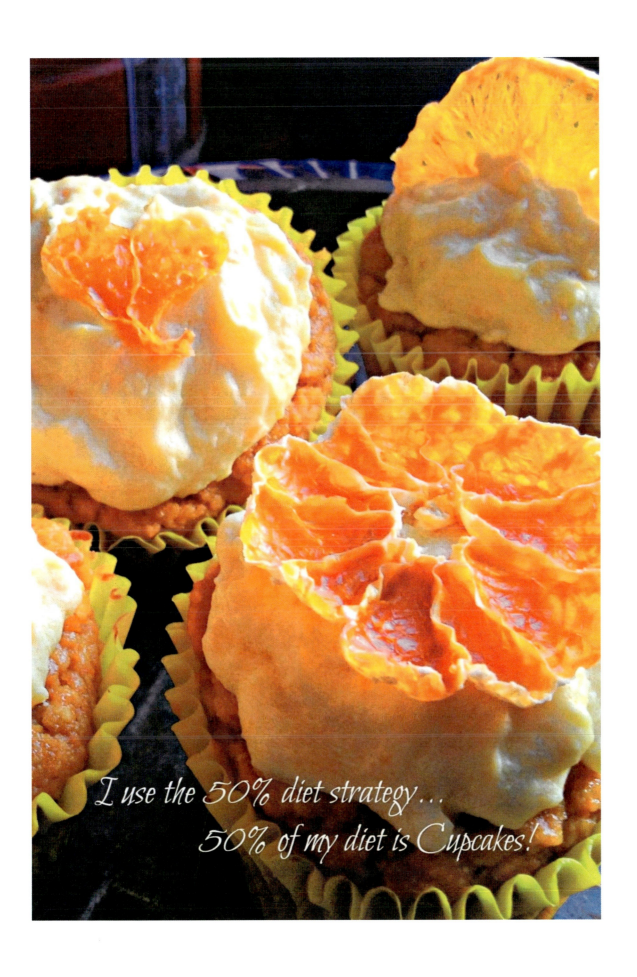

Peaches 'n Cream Cupcakes

Makes 12 Cupcakes

INGREDIENTS

1 ¼ C	Shredded Coconut
1 ¼ C	Blanched Almonds
1/2 C	Erythritol
1/2 C	Evaporated Cane Juice or 1/3 t Stevia
1 C	Chopped Sweet Potato
2 C	Chopped Peaches (about 2 Large)
3 LG	Eggs
1 T	Fresh Lemon Juice
1 T	Vanilla Extract
1 t	Almond Extract
1/2 t	Sea Salt
1 T	Egg White Powder
2 T	Coconut Flour
2 t	Baking Powder

An extra Peach for the Frosting

DIRECTIONS

Position your oven rack to lower portion of oven. Preheat the oven to 375 degrees.

Line Muffin Pan with 12 Cupcake Paper Liners. Set aside.

In your Food Processor fitted with the S Blade, add the Almonds, Coconut and Sweetener. Process for 2 or 3 minutes until it's powdery.

Add the Sweet Potato, Peaches, Lemon, Extracts and Salt. Process until smooth.

Add the Eggs and continue to process another minute until smooth and well blended.

Combine the Egg White Powder and Coconut Flour with the Baking Powder and add while the machine is running. Blend for a minute, then let set another minute.

Open the lid and check the Batter. It should be the consistency of thick pancake batter. If it is too thin, add another Tablespoon of Coconut Flour and blend again.

Using an Ice Cream Scoop or a 1/4 C measure, fill the Cupcake Liners about 3/4 full.

Bake about 12 minutes at 375, then turn the temperature down to 325 and continue baking about 25 more minutes, until a toothpick inserted comes out clean. Cover with Aluminum Foil if they begin to brown.

Cool in pans for 15 minutes, remove to finish cooling on a rack or paper towels to prevent any sogginess.

WHIPPED SWEET or COCONUT CREAM

1½ C	Heavy Whipping Cream or the 'chilled' thick Cream from a can of Coconut Milk.
2 T	Erythritol
1 t	Vanilla (optional)

Beat together with your Hand Held Mixer until thick and fluffy and soft peaks form.

Fold in 1 Peeled, Diced, Fresh Peach or Top with Sliced Peaches!

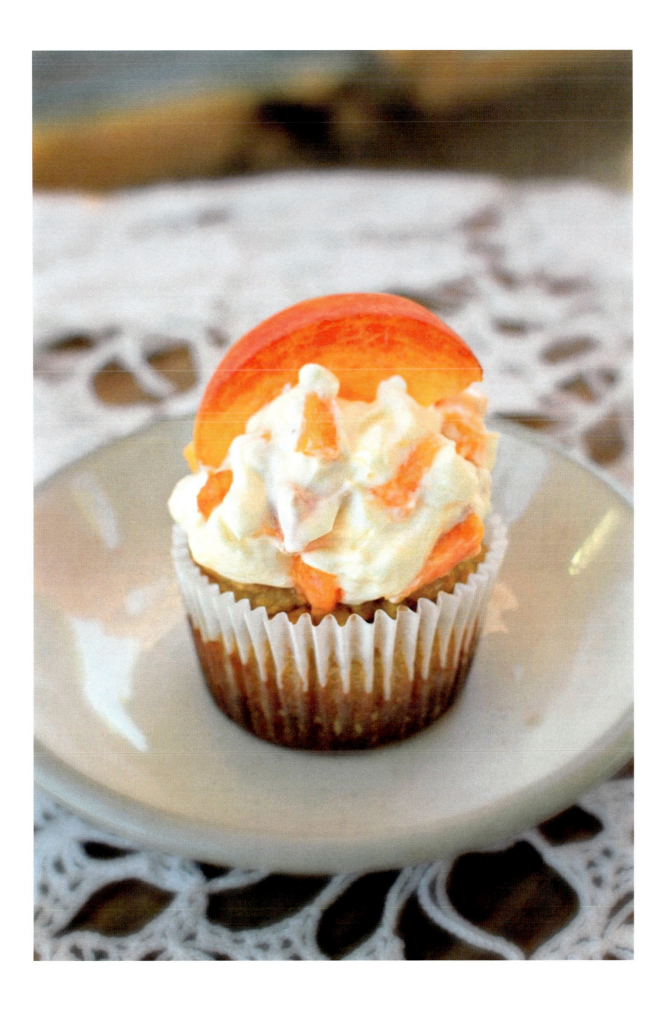

Peanut Butter 'n Jelly Cupcakes
Makes 12 Cupcakes

INGREDIENTS

1 C	Unsweetened, Shredded Coconut
1/2 C	Erythritol
1/2 C	Palm Sugar or 1/3 t Stevia
2/3 C	Peanut Butter, unsalted
1 C	Chopped Yellow Sweet Potato
1 C	Yellow Squash or peeled and chopped Zucchini (about 1 Med/LG)
1 T	Vanilla Extract
1/2 t	Sea Salt
4 LG	Eggs
2 T	Coconut Flour
2 t	Baking Powder

DIRECTIONS

Position your oven rack to lower portion of oven. Preheat the oven to 375 degrees. Line Muffin Pan with 12 Cupcake Paper Liners and set aside.

In your Food Processor fitted with the S Blade, add the Coconut and Sweetener. Process for 2 or 3 minutes until it's powdery.

Add the Sweet Potato, Zucchini or Squash, Vanilla and Salt and process until smooth.

Add the Eggs and continue to process another minute until smooth and well blended.

Combine the Coconut Flour with the Baking Powder and add while it is running. Blend for a minute, then let set another minute.

Open the lid and check the Batter. It should be the consistency of thick pancake batter. If it is too thin, add another Tablespoon of Coconut Flour and blend again.

Using an Ice Cream Scoop, fill the Cupcake Liners about 3/4 full. If possible, let the batter rest for 5-15 minutes.

Bake about 12 minutes at 375, then turn the temperature down to 325 and continue baking about 25 more minutes, until a toothpick inserted comes out clean. Cover with Aluminum Foil if they begin to brown.

Cool in pans for 15 minutes, remove to finish cooling on a rack or paper towels to prevent any sogginess.

JELLY FILLING

Press with your finger or remove a 1 inch hole in the top of the Cupcake and fill with Organic Blueberry or Grape Jam or Blend Dried Fruit with Honey to make your own.

PEANUT BUTTER FROSTING

2/3 C	Soft Butter or Palm Shortening
1/3 C	Smooth Peanut Butter
1/3 C	Maple Syrup
3 T	Baked Sweet Potato or 1 T Arrowroot
2 t	Vanilla Extract
	Pinch of Salt
	Stevia drops to taste

Blend everything together in your Food Processor until smooth.

NOTE: Buy Valencia or Jungle Peanut Butter to be safe from potential dangerous fungi. See Resources.

The only thing better than a PBJ sandwich is a PBJ Cupcake!

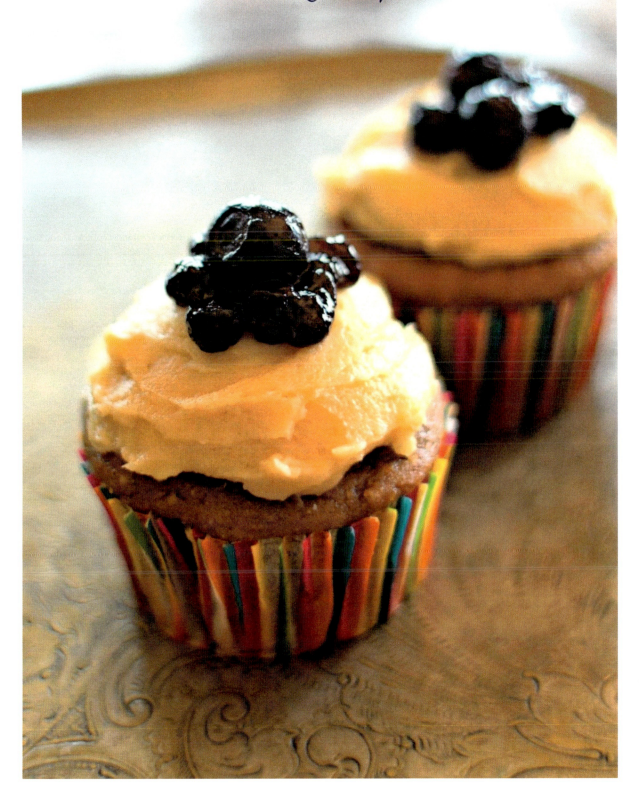

Pineapple Upside Down Cupcakes

Makes 12 Cupcakes

PINEAPPLE UPSIDE DOWN GLAZE

1 C	Chopped Pineapple
1/4 C	Palm Sugar
2-3 T	Soft Butter
6	Cherries, Fresh, cut in half

Coat the bottom and inside of each Cupcake Cup with Butter. Place half a Cherry in the center of each Cup and Sprinkle the Palm Sugar in equal portions on the bottom. Set aside.

CUPCAKE INGREDIENTS

1 1/3 C	Blanched, Slivered Almonds
1 1/3 C	Shredded, Unsweetened Coconut
1/3 C	Erythritol
1/3 C	Palm Sugar or 1/4 t Stevia
1 C	Chopped Sweet Potato
1 C	Chopped Apple (about 1 Med)
3 LG	Eggs
2 t	Vanilla Extract
1 t	Almond Extract
1/2 t	Sea Salt
1 T	Egg White Powder
2-3 T	Coconut Flour
2 t	Baking Powder

DIRECTIONS

Position your oven rack to lower/middle portion of oven. Preheat the oven to 375 degrees.

In your Food Processor fitted with the S Blade, add the Almonds, Coconut and Sweetener. Process for 2 or 3 minutes until it's powdery.

Add the Sweet Potato, Apple, Extracts and Salt and continue to process until smooth. Add the Eggs and process until smooth and well blended.

Combine the Egg White Powder and Coconut Flour with the Baking Powder and add while the machine is running. Blend for a minute then let the batter set another minute.

Open the lid and check the Batter. It should be the consistency of very thick pancake batter.

Using an Ice Cream Scoop fill the Cupcake Liners about 3/4 full.

Bake at 375 degrees for about 12 minutes, reduce the temperature to 325 degrees and continue baking until a toothpick inserted comes out clean, about another 25 minutes. Cover with Aluminum Foil if they begin to brown.

Cool in pans for 15 minutes, remove to finish cooling on a rack or paper towels to prevent any sogginess.

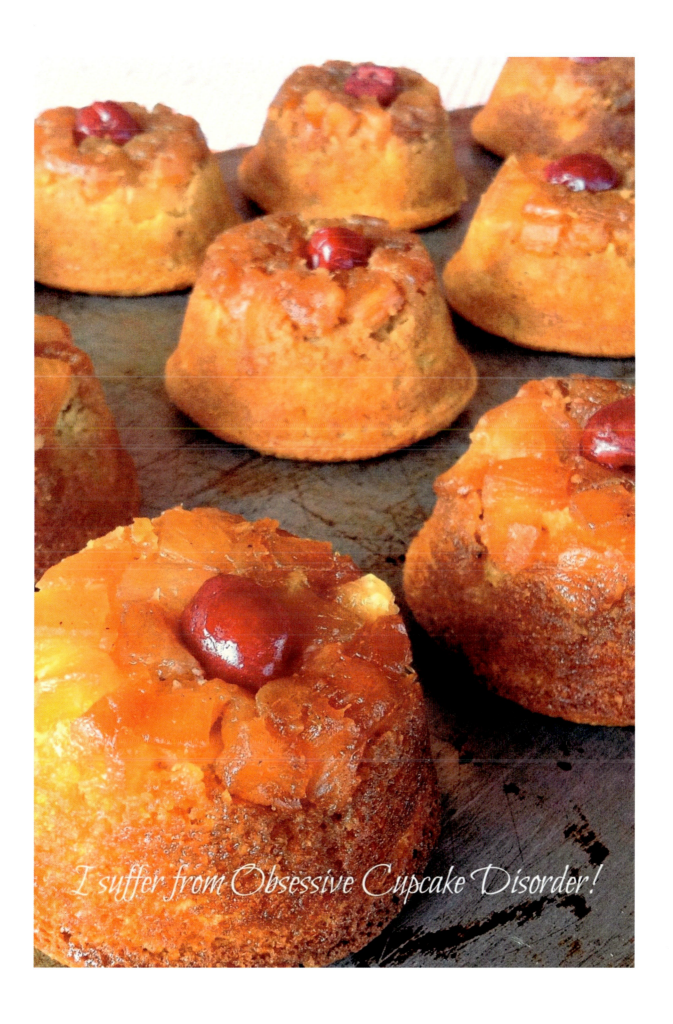

Pistachio Cupcakes
Makes 12 Cupcakes

INGREDIENTS

1 ¼ C	Blanched, Slivered Almonds
1 ¼ C	Unsweetened, Shredded Coconut
1/3 C	Raw Pistachios
1/3 C	Erythritol
1/2 C	Evaporated Cane Juice or 1/3 t Stevia
1 C	Chopped Sweet or New Potato
1 ½ C	Chopped Zucchini
3 LG	Eggs
2 t	Vanilla Extract
1/2 t	Sea Salt
1 T	Egg White Powder
2 T	Coconut Flour
2 t	Baking Powder
1/3 C	Chopped, Raw Pistachios to sprinkle on top

DIRECTIONS

Position your oven rack to lower/middle portion of oven. Preheat the oven to 400 degrees. Line Muffin Pan with 12 Cupcake Paper Liners. Set aside.

In your Food Processor fitted with the S Blade, add the Almonds, Coconut, Pistachios and Sweeteners. Process for 2 or 3 minutes until it's powdery.

Add the Potato, Zucchini, Vanilla and Salt and continue to process until smooth. Add the Eggs and process until smooth and well blended.

Combine the Egg White Powder with the Coconut Flour and Baking Powder and add while the machine is running. Blend for a minute then let the batter set another minute.

Open the lid and check the Batter. It should be the consistency of thick pancake batter.

Using an Ice Cream Scoop or a 1/4 C measure, fill the Cupcake Liners about 3/4 full.

Bake about 12 minutes at 375, then turn the temperature down to 350 and continue baking about 25-30 more minutes, until a toothpick inserted comes out clean.

Cover with Aluminum Foil if they begin to brown.

Cool in pans for 15 minutes, remove to finish cooling on a rack or paper towels to prevent sogginess.

MAGIC BUTTERCREAM FROSTING

1/2 C	Heavy Cream or Coconut/Nut Milk
1/2 C	Erythritol, Cane Sugar or Honey
1	Egg or Egg White
1/3 C	Raw, chopped Yellow Sweet Potato with skin or 2 T Arrowroot
1/2 C	Butter or Palm Shortening
2 t	Vanilla Extract
1/4 t	Guar Gum
1/8 t	Sea Salt
	Stevia drops to taste

Combine all ingredients, *except* the Shortening or Butter, in your blender and blend until very smooth.

Strain into a small saucepan and while stirring, bring the mixture to a simmer until it's thickened.

Stir in the Butter or Shortening until melted and transfer the mixture to the bowl of your Stand Mixer.

Chill until cold then beat several minutes until fluffy.

TIP: You can also let the mixture cool to room temperature and add the Butter or Shortening a little at a time while beating until fluffy.

NOTE: The frosting will be cream colored or whiter depending upon the ingredients used.

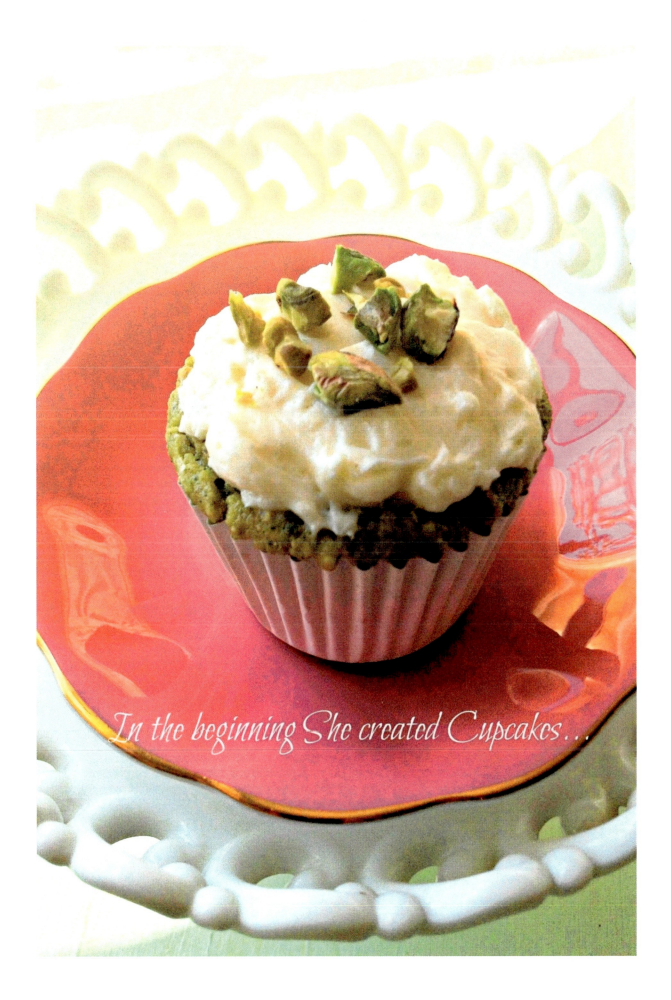

Red Velvet Cupcakes

Makes 12 Cupcakes

INGREDIENTS

1 ¼ C	Blanched, Slivered Almonds
1 ¼ C	Shredded, Unsweetened Coconut
1/2 C	Erythritol
1/2 C	Evaporated Cane Sugar or 1/3 t Stevia
1 C	Chopped Sweet or New Potato
1 C	Rough Chopped, Peeled, Raw Beet
1 C	Pitted Cherries (previously frozen is fine)
3 LG	Eggs
1 T	Lemon Juice
2 T	Vanilla Extract
1 t	Almond Extract
1/2 t	Sea Salt
1 T	Egg White Powder
3 T	Coconut Flour
2 t	Baking Powder
2 T	Cocoa Powder (optional)

DIRECTIONS

Position your oven rack to lower portion of oven. Preheat the oven to 375 degrees. Line Muffin Pan with 12 Cupcake Paper Liners. Set aside.

In your Food Processor fitted with the S Blade, add the Almonds, Coconut and Sweetener. Process for 2 or 3 minutes until it's powdery.

Add the Sweet or New Potato, Beet, Cherries and Lemon Juice and Process until smooth.

Add the Eggs, Extracts and Salt and continue to process another minute until smooth and well blended.

Combine the Egg White Powder and Coconut Flour with the Baking Powder and add while the machine is running. Blend for a minute then let the batter set another minute.

Open the lid and check the Batter. It should be the consistency of thick pancake batter. If it seems too thin add another Tablespoon of Coconut Flour and blend again.

Using an Ice Cream Scoop fill the Cupcake Liners about 3/4 full.

Bake at 375 degrees for about 12 minutes, reduce the temperature to 325 degrees and continue baking until a toothpick inserted comes out clean, about another 25 minutes. Cover with Aluminum Foil if they begin to brown.

Cool in pan for 15 minutes, then transfer to a wire rack to finish cooling before frosting.

FLUFFY CREAM CHEESE FROSTING

1/2 C	Cream Cheese
1/2 C	Powdered Sugar or Erythritol
1 t	Vanilla Extract
1/2 t	Almond Extract
1/2 C	Heavy Cream
	Stevia drops to taste

With an electric mixer on medium speed, whip the Cream Cheese until creamy. Add the Sweetener, Extracts and half of the Cream and beat until smooth. Gradually add the rest of the Cream. Chill until very cold then whip on high until stiff.

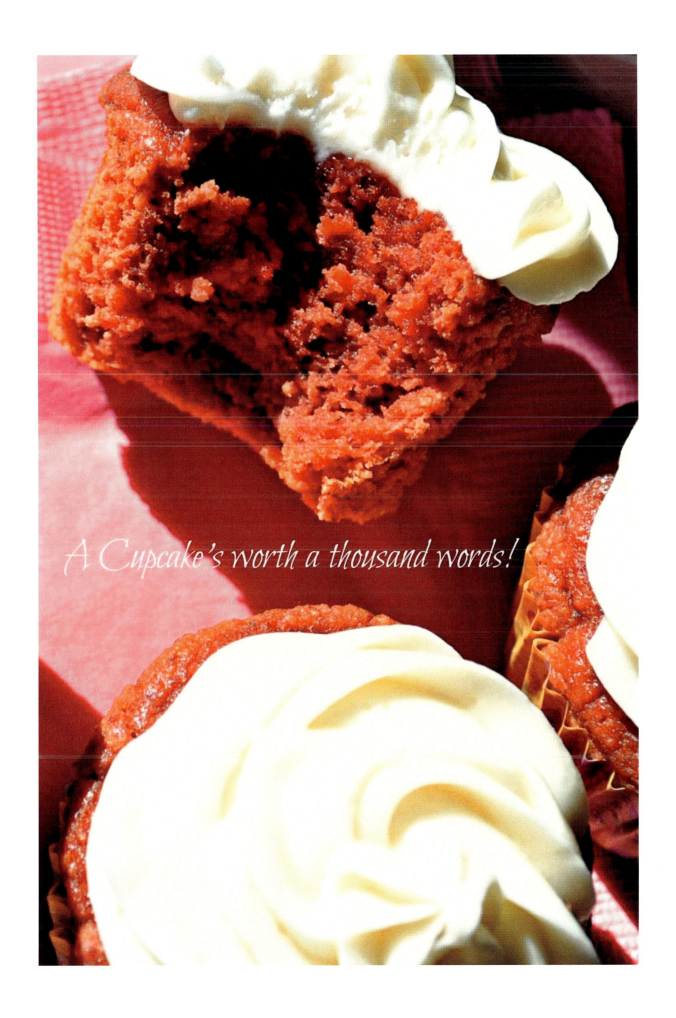

Rich White Cupcakes
Makes 12 Cupcakes

INGREDIENTS

1 ¼ C	Blanched, Slivered Almonds
1 ¼ C	Shredded, Unsweetened Coconut
1/3 C	Erythritol
1/2 C	Evaporated Cane Juice or 1/3 t Stevia
2/3 C	Chopped, Peeled New Potatoes
1/3 C	Heavy Cream or Coconut Milk
4 LG	Egg Whites
2 T	Vanilla Extract
2 t	Lemon Juice
1 t	Almond Extract
1/2 t	Sea Salt
1 T	Egg White Powder
3 T	Coconut Flour
2 t	Baking Powder

DIRECTIONS

Position your oven rack to lower portion of oven. Preheat the oven to 375 degrees. Line Muffin Pan with 12 Cupcake Paper Liners and set aside.

In your Food Processor fitted with the S Blade, add the Almonds, Coconut and Sweetener. Process for 2 or 3 minutes until it's powdery.

Add the Potatoes, Heavy Cream or Coconut Milk and process until smooth. Add the Eggs, Extracts, Lemon Juice and Salt and continue to process another minute until smooth and well blended.

Combine the Coconut Flour with the Baking Powder and add while the machine is running. Blend for a minute then let the batter set another minute.

Open the lid and check the Batter. It should be the consistency of very thick pancake batter. Using an Ice Cream Scoop, fill the Cupcake Liners about 3/4 full.

Bake at 375 degrees for about 12 minutes.

Reduce the temperature to 325 degrees and continue baking until a toothpick comes out clean, about another 25 minutes. Cover with Aluminum Foil if they begin to brown.

Cool in pans for 15 minutes, remove to finish cooling on a rack or paper towels to prevent sogginess.

TIP: You can replace the Cream and Lemon Juice with Sour Cream.

TIP: Use the egg yolks in ice cream, smoothies, or give them to your favorite dog or cat!

Frost with: **MAGIC BUTTERCREAM** page 136 or

FLUFFY WHITE FROSTING

1/2 C	Palm Shortening
1/2 C	Powdered Sugar or Erythritol plus 1 T Arrowroot
2 T	Sour Cream
1 t	Vanilla Extract
1/2 t	Almond Extract
1/8 t	Guar Gum
	Pinch of Sea Salt
1/2 C	Heavy Cream
	Stevia drops to taste

With an electric mixer on medium speed, blend all of the ingredients until creamy. Chill until very cold then beat until fluffy.

NOTE: *Erythritol will re-crystallize and give the frosting a nice 'crunch' that kids love. If you don't want that crunch use all Powdered Sugar.

TIP: To make this frosting Vegan, omit the Sour Cream and replace the Heavy Cream with Heavy Coconut Cream (the heavy coconut cream from the top of the chilled can.

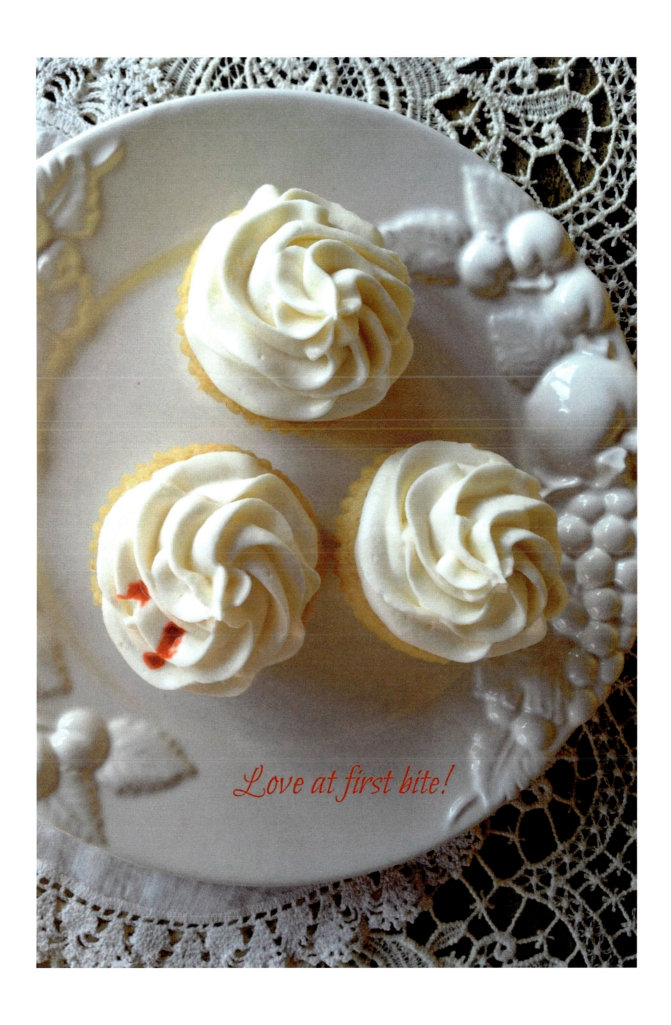

S'morelicious Cupcakes

Makes 12 Cupcakes

INGREDIENTS

1 C	Shredded Coconut
1 C	Blanched Almonds
2/3 C	Walnuts or Pecans
1/2 C	Palm Sugar
1/2 C	Erythritol
1 C	Chopped Sweet Potato
1 ½ C	Chopped Tomatoes (about 2 medium)
3 LG	Eggs plus 1 Yolk
1 T	Vanilla Extract
1/2 t	Cinnamon
1/2 t	Sea Salt
1/2 t	Espresso Powder
1 T	Egg White Powder
2 T	Coconut Flour
2 t	Baking Powder
1/3 C	Chocolate Chips

DIRECTIONS

Position your oven rack to lower portion of oven. Preheat the oven to 375 degrees.

Line Muffin Pan with 12 Cupcake Paper Liners. Set aside.

In your Food Processor fitted with the S Blade, add the Almonds, Walnuts or Pecans, Coconut and Sweetener. Process for 2 or 3 minutes until it's powdery.

Add the Sweet Potato, Tomatoes, Vanilla, Cinnamon, Salt and Espresso Powder, process until smooth.

Add the Eggs and continue to process another minute until smooth and well blended.

Combine the Egg White Powder and Coconut Flour with the Baking Powder and add while the machine is running. Blend for a minute, then let set another minute.

Open the lid and check the Batter. It should be the consistency of thick pancake batter. If it is too thin, add another Tablespoon of Coconut Flour and blend. Using an Ice Cream Scoop or a 1/4 C measure, fill the Cupcake Liners about 3/4 full.

Press 5-7 Chocolate Chips into the center of the Cupcake batter.

Bake about 12 minutes at 375, then turn the temperature down to 325 and continue baking about another 25 more minutes, until a toothpick comes out clean. Cover with Aluminum Foil if they begin to brown.

TOASTED MARSHMALLOW FROSTING

1 LG	Egg White (use yolk in Filling above)
1/3 C	Palm Sugar
2 T	Maple Syrup
1 ½ T	Water
1/8 t	Cream of Tartar
1/8 t	Sea Salt
1 t	Vanilla Extract

Combine all the ingredients except the Extracts in a Double Boiler (or use a Tall Stainless Bowl set on a pan of Boiling Water-don't let the bottom of the pan touch the water).

Beat with your Hand Held Mixer for 6 minutes. It will become light and creamy and triple in size.

Remove the bowl from the heat, add the Extracts and beat 1 more minute.

TIP: Add 1/8 t Guar Gum to frosting if you plan to freeze these.

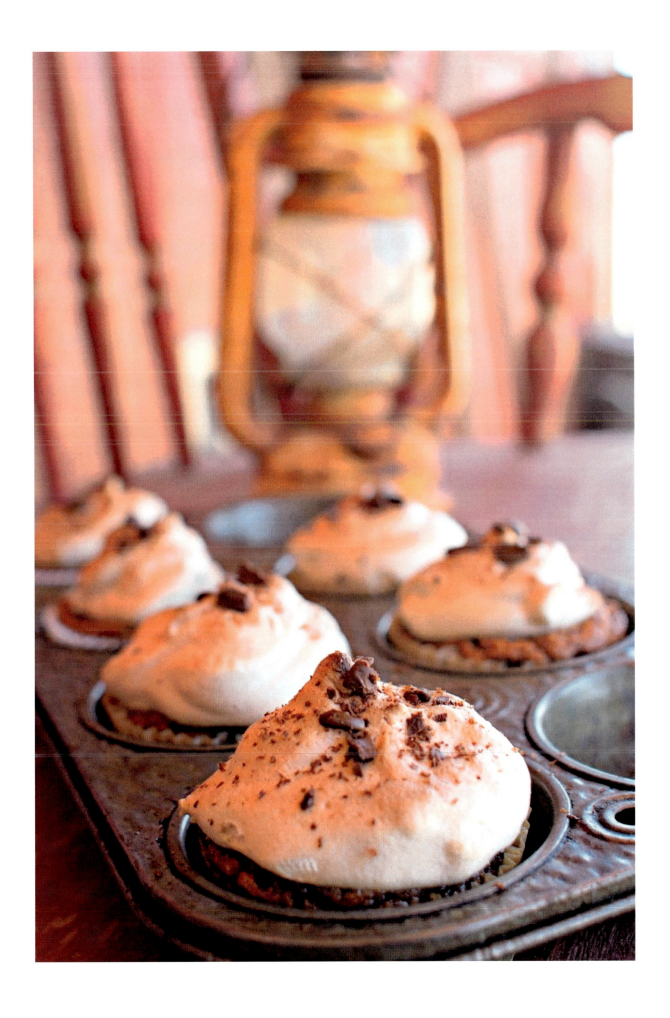

Strawberry Shortcake Cupcakes
Makes 12 Cupcakes

INGREDIENTS

1 1/3 C	Blanched, Slivered Almonds
1 1/3 C	Shredded, Unsweetened Coconut
1/3 C	Honey
1/3 C	Erythritol
1 C	Chopped Yellow Sweet Potato
4 LG	Eggs
1 T	Lemon Juice
1 t	Vanilla Extract
1/2 t	Sea Salt
1 T	Egg White Powder
1-2 T	Coconut Flour
2 t	Baking Powder
1 1/3 C	Diced Strawberries
	A few Sliced Strawberries for Decoration

DIRECTIONS

Position your oven rack to lower portion of oven. Preheat the oven to 375 degrees. Line Muffin Pan with 12 Cupcake Paper Liners and set aside.

In your Food Processor fitted with the S Blade, add the Almonds, Coconut and Sweetener. Process for 2 or 3 minutes until it's powdery.

Add the Sweet Potato, Lemon Juice, Vanilla, and Salt and process until smooth, add the Eggs and continue to process another minute until smooth and well blended.

Combine the Egg White Powder and Coconut Flour with the Baking Powder and add while the machine is running.

Blend for a minute then let the batter set another minute.

Open the lid and check the Batter. It should be the consistency of thick pancake batter. Stir in the Diced Fruit.

Using an Ice Cream Scoop, fill the Cupcake Liners about 3/4 full.

Bake at 375 degrees for about 12 minutes, reduce the temperature to 325 degrees and continue baking until a toothpick comes out clean, about another 25 minutes. Cover with Aluminum Foil if they begin to brown.

Cool in pans for 15 minutes, remove to finish cooling on a rack or paper towels to prevent any sogginess.

SWEET WHIPPED CREAM FROSTING

1 ½ C	Heavy Cream
2 T	Powdered Sugar
1 t	Vanilla extract

Whip with hand held mixer until soft peaks form.

VARIATION: Crush the Strawberries with a little Sweetener and a pinch of Guar Gum. Cut out the center of the Cupcakes, fill with the Macerated Strawberries and top with the Cream and a Fresh Berry.

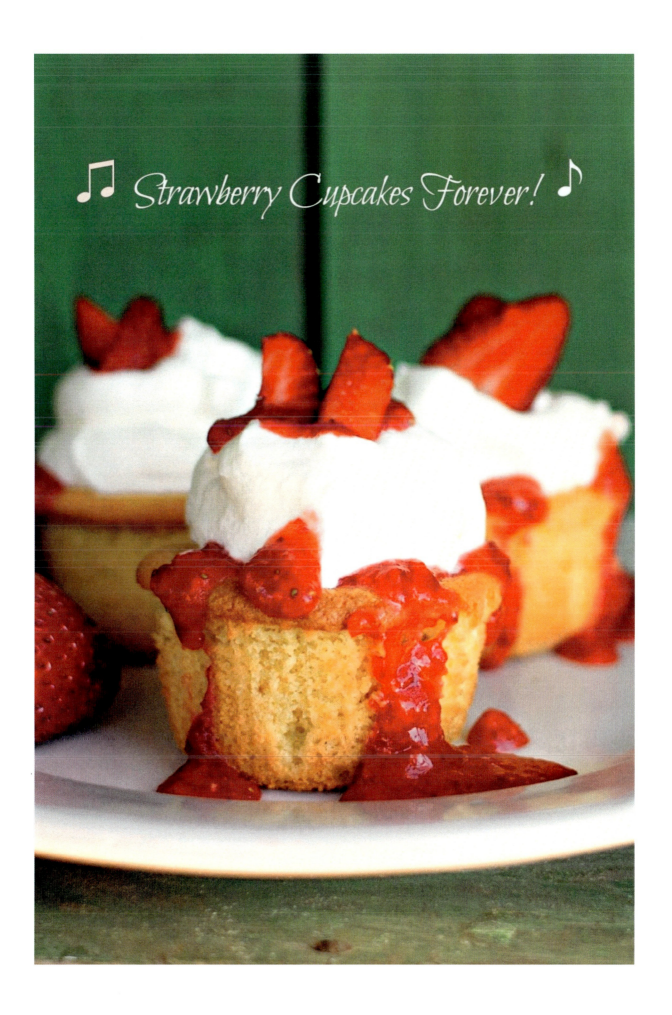

Tiramisu Cupcakes
Makes 12 Cupcakes

INGREDIENTS

1 ¼ C	Blanched, Slivered Almonds
1 ¼ C	Unsweetened, Shredded Coconut
1/2 C	Erythritol
1/2 C	Palm Sugar or 1/3 t Stevia
1 C	Chopped New Potato
2/3 C	Chopped, peeled Zucchini
4 LG	Eggs
1 T	Vanilla Extract
1 T	Ground Instant Espresso Powder
1/2 t	Sea Salt
1 T	Egg White Powder
1-2 T	Coconut Flour
1 T	Baking Powder

DIRECTIONS

Position your oven rack to lower portion of oven. Preheat the oven to 400 degrees. Line Muffin Pan with 12 Cupcake Paper Liners and set aside.

In your Food Processor fitted with the S Blade, add the Almonds, Coconut and Sweetener. Process for 2 or 3 minutes until it's powdery.

Add the Potato, Zucchini, Vanilla and Salt. Continue to process. Add the Eggs and process until smooth.

Combine the Egg White Powder and Coconut Flour with the Baking Powder and add while the machine is running, blend, then let the batter set a minute.

Open the lid and check the Batter. It should be the consistency of thick pancake batter. If it's thinner, blend in another Tablespoon of Coconut Flour.

Using an Ice Cream Scoop, fill the Cupcake Liners about 3/4 full.

Bake about 12 minutes at 375 degrees, then turn the oven down to 325 and continue baking about another 25 minutes, until a toothpick comes out clean. Cover with Aluminum Foil if they begin to brown.

Cool in pans for 15 minutes, remove to finish cooling on a rack or paper towels to prevent any sogginess.

While the Cupcakes are Baking and Cooling...

SYRUP

1/3 C	Strong Hot Coffee or Espresso
2 T	Palm Sugar or Maple Syrup
2 T	Rum

Stir together until the Sweetener is dissolved.

FILLING

1 ½ C	Mascarpone Cheese
2/3 C	Powdered Palm Sugar
2 T	Rum
2 T	Strong Coffee or Espresso
2 T	Cocoa Powder

Blend together until smooth.

FLUFFY TOPPING

Leftover Filling from above *(after you have filled the hole you made in the Cupcake with the Filling there should be about 1 C left)*

1 C	Heavy Cream, whipped to stiff peaks
1 t	Powdered Instant Espresso (optional)
	Maple Syrup or Stevia drops to your taste

Stir all together.

TO ASSEMBLE

Once the Cupcakes have cooled cut off the tops with a sharp knife. Lay them upside down next to the Cupcakes. Now, cut out a small hole in the Cupcake less than an inch wide and deep.

Brush the Cupcake and the upside down top with the Syrup. Coat both well, at least two times but don't use quite all the Syrup. Next, fill the holes with a teaspoon of the Filling.

Now, spoon about 2 T of the Fluffy Topping onto the Cupcake over the Filling. Put the cut off top on top of the Fluffy Topping right-side up. Top with more of the Fluffy Topping and dust with Cocoa Powder.

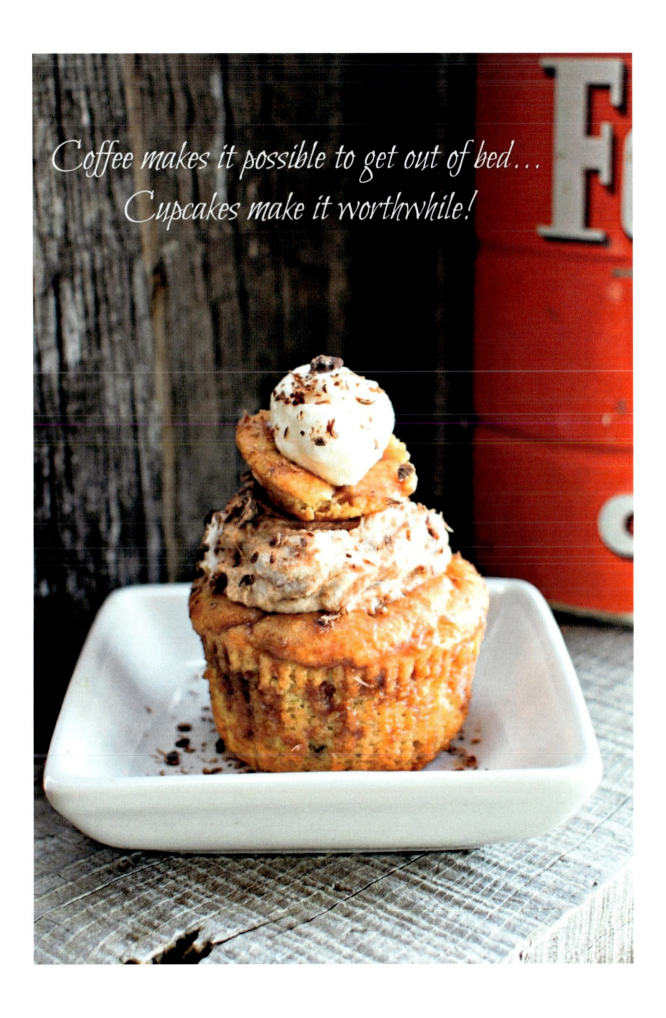

Very Vanilla Cupcakes

Makes 12 Cupcakes

INGREDIENTS

1 ½ C	Blanched, Slivered Almonds
1 C	Shredded, Unsweetened Coconut
1/2 C	Erythritol
1/2 C	Evaporated Cane Sugar or 1/3 t Stevia
1 C	Chopped Sweet Potato
1 ½ C	Peeled and Chopped Zucchini or Yellow Squash (about 1 Med/LG)
3 LG	Eggs
2 T	Vanilla Extract or Paste
2 t	Lemon Juice
1 t	Almond Extract
1/2 t	Sea Salt
1 T	Egg White Powder
2-3 T	Coconut Flour
2 t	Baking Powder

DIRECTIONS

Position your oven rack to middle/lower portion of oven.

Preheat the oven to 375 degrees. Line Muffin Pan with 12 Cupcake Paper Liners and set aside.

In your Food Processor fitted with the S Blade, add the Almonds, Coconut and Sweetener. Process for 2 or 3 minutes until it's powdery.

Add the Sweet Potato, Zucchini or Squash, Extracts, Lemon Juice and Salt and continue to process until smooth. Add the Eggs and process until smooth and well blended.

Combine the Egg White Powder and Coconut Flour with the Baking Powder and add while the machine is running. Blend for a minute then let the batter set another minute.

Open the lid and check the Batter. It should be the consistency of thick pancake batter.

Using an Ice Cream Scoop, fill the Cupcake Liners about 3/4 full.

Bake at 375 degrees about 12 minutes, reduce the temperature to 325 degrees and continue baking until a toothpick comes out clean, about another 25 minutes. Cover with Aluminum Foil if they begin to brown.

Cool in pans for 15 minutes, remove to finish cooling on a rack or paper towels to prevent any sogginess.

Frost with: **MAGIC BUTTERCREAM** page 136 or

CREAMY VANILLA FROSTING

1/2 C	Palm Shortening
1/4 C	Maple Syrup
1/4 C	Erythritol or Powdered Sugar
3 T	Baked Sweet Potato or 2 T Arrowroot
1 T	Vanilla Paste or Extract
1/8 t	Guar Gum
1/2 C	Heavy Cream or Heavy Coconut Cream (from the top of the chilled can)

Cream all together in your Food Processor, chill until very cold and whip until fluffy.

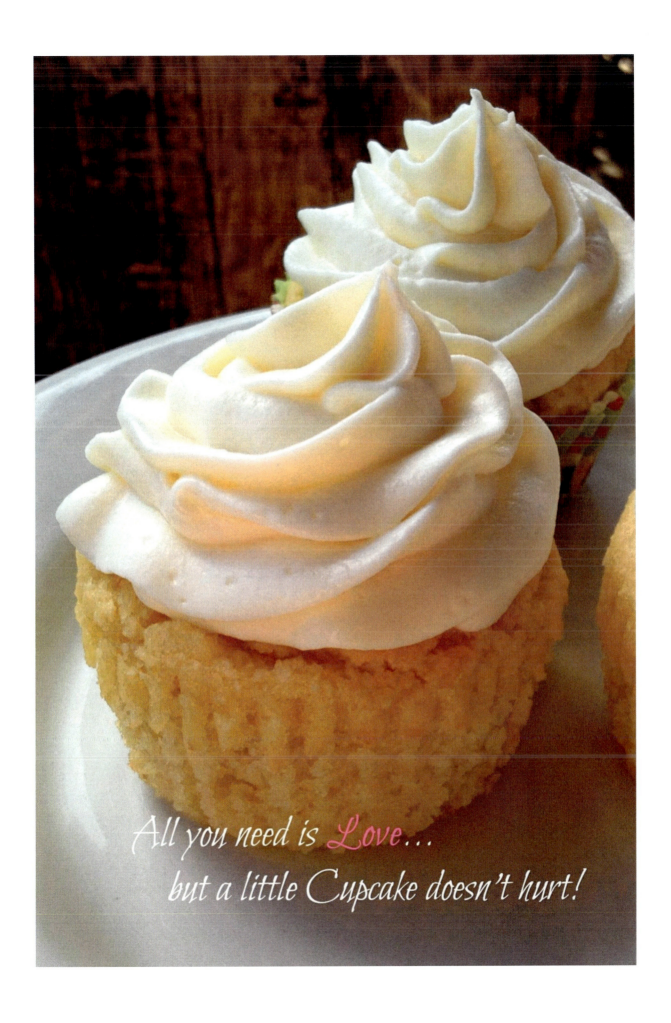

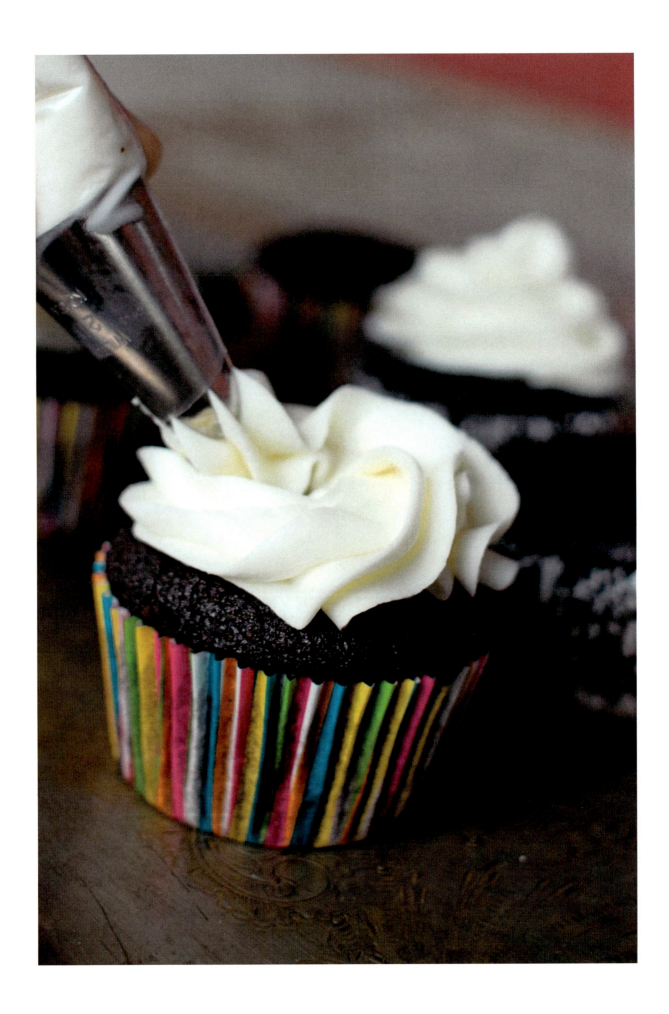

FROSTINGS

Brown Buttercream	106
Buttery Cream Cheese	107
Coconut Lime Cream Cheese	108
Coconut Pecan	109
Creamy Vanilla	110
Dark Chocolate or Vanilla Buttercream	111
Fluffy Chocolate	112
Fluffy Cream Cheese	113
Fluffy Raspberry	114
Fluffy White	115
Magic Buttercream	116
Milk Chocolate	117
Orange Cream	118
Peanut Butter	119
Sweet Whipped or Coconut Cream	120
White Chocolate Cream	120
7 Minute Meringue	121

SWEET SAUCES

Dark Coconut Palm Caramel Sauce	122
Easy Chocolate Sauce	122

NOTE: Some of these recipes give the option of using either Powdered Sugar or Erythritol. Erythritol will re-crystallize and give the frosting a nice 'crunch' that kids and many adults love. If you don't want that crunch, use Powdered Sugar. I often use half of each, which adds just a little 'crunch'! If a sweeter frosting is desired, a drop or two of Stevia works perfectly!

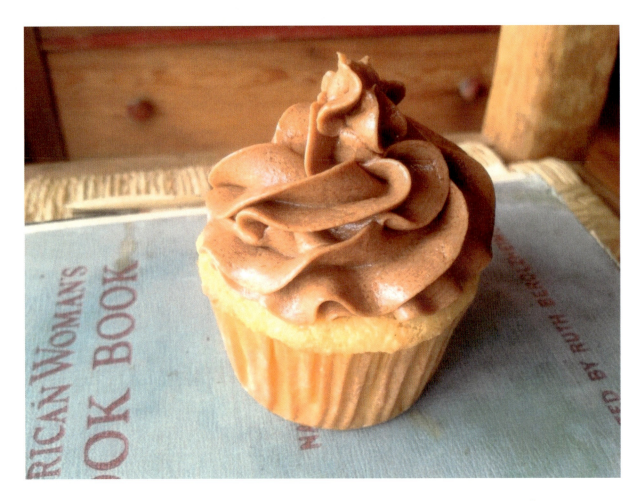

Brown Buttercream Frosting
Frosts 12 Cupcakes

1 C	Softened, unsalted Butter
1/2 C	Maple Syrup *or* Honey
3 T	Baked Sweet Potato *or* 2 T Arrowroot Powder
2 t	Vanilla Extract
1/8 t	Guar Gum
2 T	Palm Sugar (optional, for a darker frosting)
	Pinch of Sea Salt

Blend all in your 4 C Food Processor until fluffy.

TIP: For more sweetness add a drop or two of Stevia.
TIP: Guar Gum helps to make a fluffy frosting, but its use is optional!

Buttery Cream Cheese Frosting
Frosts 12 Cupcakes

1/2 C	Cream Cheese
1/2 C	Soft Butter
1/2 C	Powdered Sugar *or* Erythritol
1/2 t	Vanilla Extract
	Pinch of Sea Salt
	Stevia drops to taste

In your Food Processor or with a Handheld Mixer whip the Cream Cheese until smooth.

Add the Butter and blend well.

Add the Sweetener, Vanilla and Salt and beat 'til smooth.

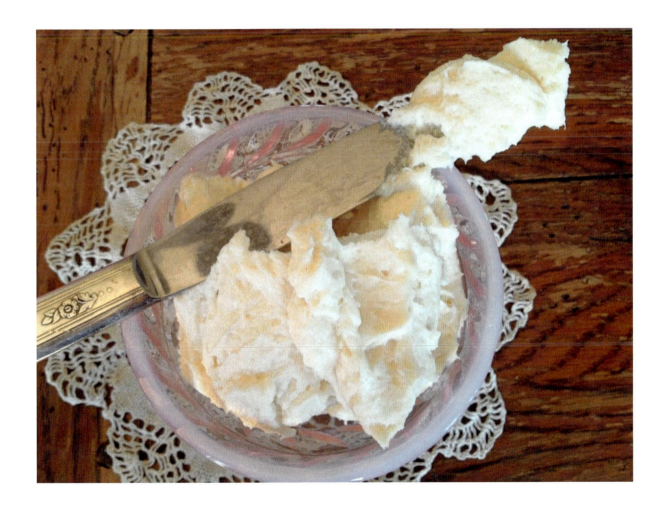

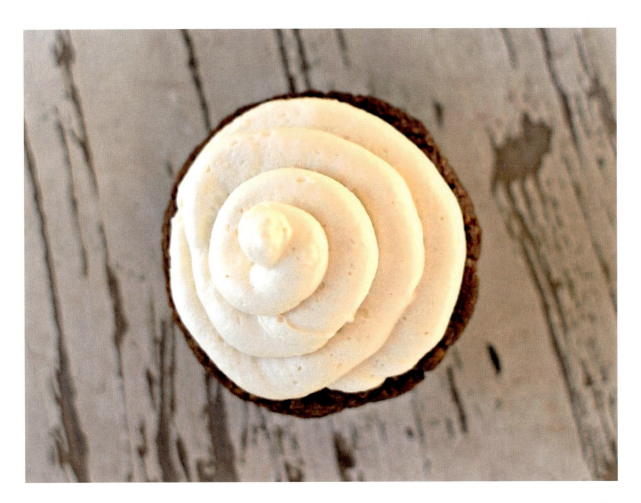

Coconut Lime Cream Cheese Frosting
Frosts 12 Cupcakes

1/2 C	Softened Cream Cheese
1/3 C	Coconut Cream *or* Heavy Cream
2-3 T	Coconut Oil, melted
1/2 C	Powdered Sugar *or* Erythritol
1 t	Vanilla Extract
	Zest of 1/2 a Lime
	Stevia drops to taste

Blend the Cream Cheese with Coconut Cream or Heavy Cream until smooth. Pour in the Coconut Oil while blending. Add the rest of the ingredients and blend again until smooth.

Chill in Refrigerator until cold then whip until Fluffy.

Frost the cooled Cupcakes and sprinkle with the end of the Lime Zest.

Coconut Pecan Frosting
Frosts 12 Cupcakes

2	Egg Yolks
3/4 C	Heavy Cream *or* Coconut/Nut Milk
1/3 C	Erythritol
1/3 C	Palm Sugar *or* Maple Syrup
1 C	Chopped Pecans
3/4 C	Shredded, unsweetened Coconut
1/4 C	Coconut Oil
	Stevia drops to taste

Blend Egg Yolks, Cream or Coconut Milk and Sweetener together in a saucepan. Simmer about 5 minutes until thick. Remove from heat and stir in the rest of the ingredients. Cool a bit, but frost while still warm.

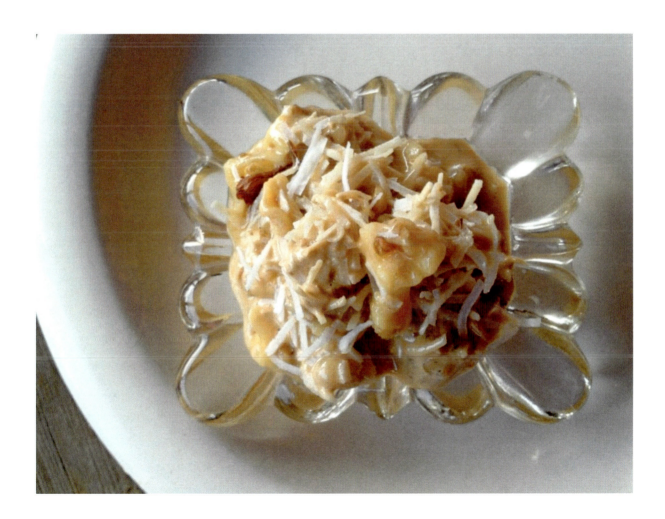

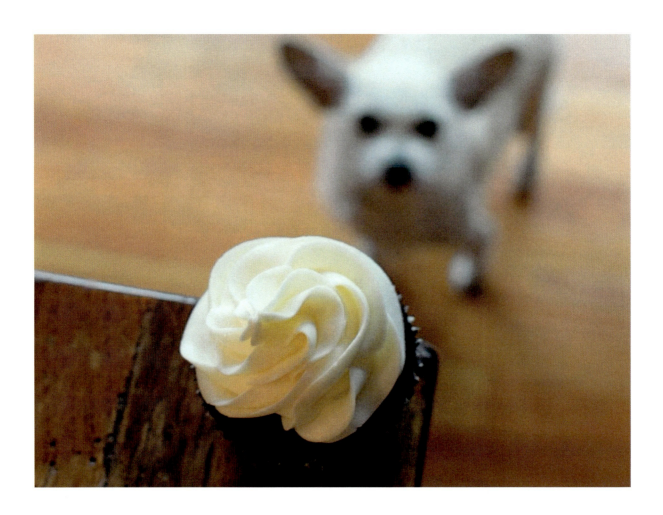

Creamy Vanilla Frosting
Frosts 12 Cupcakes

1/2 C	Palm Shortening
1/4 C	Maple Syrup
1/4 C	Erythritol *or* Powdered Sugar
3 T	Baked Sweet Potato *or* 2 T Arrowroot Powder
1 T	Vanilla Extract *or* Paste (the paste or fresh bean gives nice vanilla 'specks')
1/8 t	Guar Gum
1/2 C	Heavy Cream *or* Heavy Coconut Cream (from the top of the chilled can)
	Stevia drops to taste

Cream all together in your Food Processor, chill if necessary & whip until fluffy.

Dark Chocolate Buttercream
Frosts 12 Cupcakes

2 LG	Egg Whites
2/3 C	Erythritol *or* Evaporated Cane Sugar *or* Honey
1/2 C	Butter *or* Palm Shortening
1/2 C	Bittersweet Chocolate, melted and cooled
2 t	Vanilla Extract
1 t	Espresso powder (optional)
	Pinch of Sea Salt
	Stevia Drops to taste, 2-4

Combine the Eggs, Sweetener and Salt in the Stainless Steel Bowl of your Stand Mixer and set on top of a saucepan of simmering water on your stove. Whisk for a few minutes until the Sweetener has dissolved and the Eggs are quite warm. Transfer bowl to your Mixer and beat on medium speed for several minutes until cooled and stiff peaks form. Add the Butter or Palm Shortening a little at a time and beat until smooth. Add Vanilla, Espresso and the cooled Chocolate. Blend until combined, increase the speed and beat until fluffy. **TIP:** If the frosting is too warm, chill and beat again!

FOR VANILLA: Omit the Chocolate and Espresso and decrease the Sweetener to 1/2 Cup.

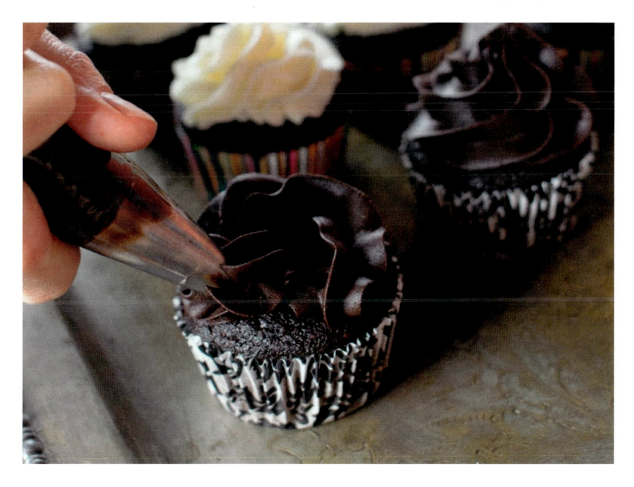

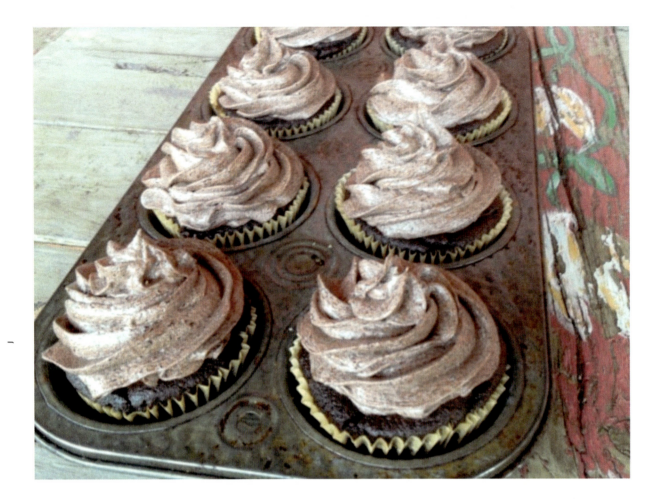

Fluffy Chocolate Frosting
Frosts 12 Cupcakes

1 C	Soft Butter *or* Palm Shortening
1/3 C	Cocoa Powder (Raw Cacao is best!)
1/2 C	Powdered Sugar *or* Erythritol
2 t	Vanilla Extract
1 t	Almond Extract
1/8 t	Sea Salt
	Pinch of Guar Gum
	Stevia drops to taste

Blend the Butter with the Cocoa until smooth. Add the Sweetener and other ingredients and blend until creamy.

Chill before frosting Cupcakes.

TIP: You may substitute the Butter with Palm Shortening or even a 'just ripe' Avocado!

Fluffy Cream Cheese Frosting
Frosts 12 Cupcakes

1/2 C	Cream Cheese
1/2 C	Powdered Sugar *or* Erythritol
1 t	Vanilla Extract
1/2 t	Almond Extract
1/2 C	Heavy Cream
	Stevia drops to taste

Using your Handheld Mixer, whip the Cream Cheese until smooth.

Add the Sweetener, Extracts and half the Cream and beat 'til smooth.

Continue beating while you gradually add the rest of the Cream.

Refrigerate until very cold and beat until fluffy.

VARIATION: Grind 1/2 C of freeze dried fruit, such as strawberries, in your coffee grinder to a fine powder. Whip into the mixture to create a Strawberry Cream Cheese Frosting.

TIP: If you are out of Heavy Cream you may adjust the recipe by increasing the Cream Cheese to 1 C and substituting the Cream for 1/4 C of Water or Coconut/Almond Milk.

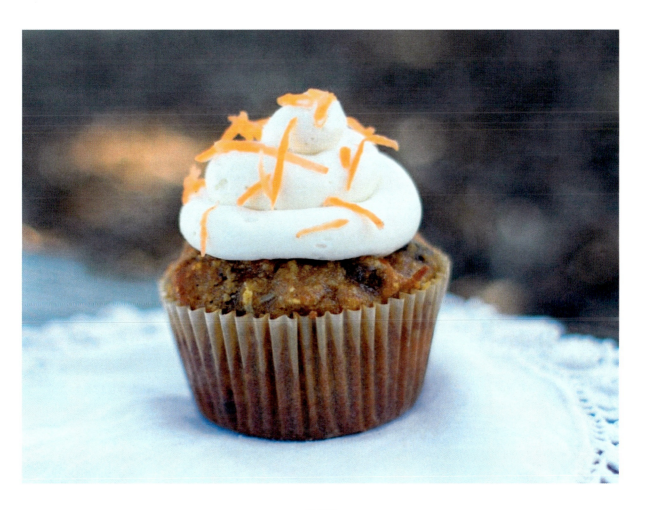

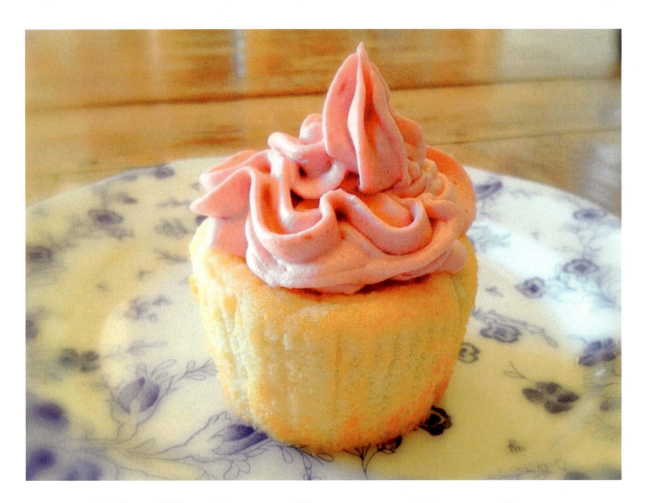

Fluffy Raspberry Frosting
Frosts 12 Cupcakes

1/2 C	Palm Shortening	
2/3 C	Powdered Sugar *or* Erythritol	
1 C	Freeze-dried Raspberries powdered in your Coffee Grinder	
2 t	Vanilla Extract	
1/2 t	Almond Extract	
1/8 t	Guar Gum	
	Pinch of Sea Salt	
1/2 C	Heavy Cream	
	Stevia drops to taste	

With an electric mixer on medium speed, blend all of the ingredients until creamy. Chill until very cold then beat until fluffy.

TIP: You can make this any Fruit Flavor you want by simply changing the Freeze-dried Fruit you choose!

TIP: To make this frosting Vegan, replace the Heavy Cream with Heavy Coconut Cream (the heavy coconut cream from the top of the chilled can).

Fluffy White Frosting
Frosts 12 Cupcakes

1/2 C	Palm Shortening
1/2 C	Powdered Sugar *or* Erythritol *plus* 2 T Arrowroot
2 T	Sour Cream
1 t	Vanilla Extract
1/2 t	Almond Extract
1/8 t	Guar Gum
	Pinch of Sea Salt
1/2 C	Heavy Cream

With an electric mixer on medium speed, blend all of the ingredients until creamy.

Chill until very cold then beat until fluffy.

TIP: For a sweeter frosting add Stevia drops to taste.

TIP: To make this frosting Vegan, omit the Sour Cream and replace the Heavy Cream with Heavy Coconut Cream (Heavy Coconut Cream from the top of the chilled can).

NOTE: Remember, if you use Erythritol the frosting will have a nice little 'crunch'!

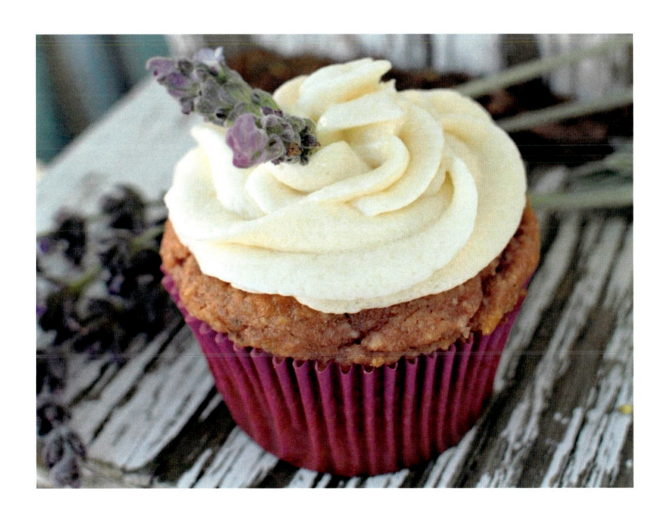

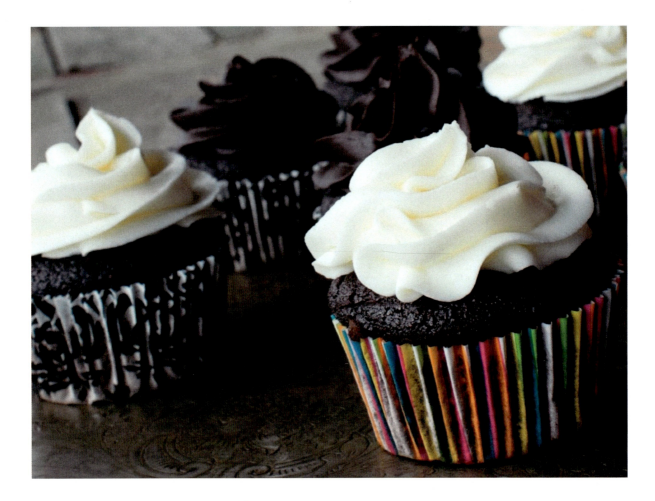

Magic Buttercream
Frosts 12 Cupcakes

1/2 C	Cream *or* Coconut/Almond Milk
1/2 C	Erythritol, Evaporated Cane Sugar *or* Honey,
1	Egg *or* Egg White
1/3 C	Raw, chopped Sweet Potato with skin *or* 2 T Arrowroot
1/2 C	Butter *or* Palm Shortening
1 t	Vanilla Extract
1/4 t	Guar Gum
1/8 t	Sea Salt
	Stevia Drops to taste

Combine all ingredients *except* the Shortening or Butter in a blender and blend until smooth.

Strain into a small saucepan and, while stirring constantly, bring the mixture to a simmer until it's thickened.

Stir in the Butter or Shortening until melted and transfer the mixture to the bowl of your Stand Mixer. Chill until cold then beat several minutes until fluffy.

TIP: You can also let the mixture cool to room temperature and add the Butter or Shortening a little at a time while beating until fluffy.

NOTE: The frosting will be cream colored or whiter depending upon the ingredients used.

CHOCOLATE: Increase the Sweetener to 2/3 C and stir into the hot, thickened mixture 1/3 C Bittersweet Chocolate pieces.

CARAMEL: Replace Sweetener with Palm Sugar and add 1/8 t Baking Soda to Blender.

Milk Chocolate Frosting
Frosts 12 Cupcakes

1/2 C	Palm Shortening	
2 T	Baked Sweet Potato *or* 1 T Arrowroot	
3 T	Cocoa Powder (Raw Cacao is best)	
1/3 C	Maple Syrup	
3 T	Erythritol *or* Palm Sugar	
1 t	Vanilla Extract	
	Pinch of Guar Gum	
	Pinch of Sea Salt	
1/2 C	Heavy Cream *or* Heavy Coconut Cream (from the top of the chilled can)	

Blend the Shortening, Sweet Potato or Arrowroot and Cocoa Powder in your 4 Cup Food Processor 'til creamy.

Add the rest of the ingredients, **except** the Heavy Cream, and blend until very smooth.

Chill if necessary. Add the Heavy Cream slowly and whip 'til fluffy.

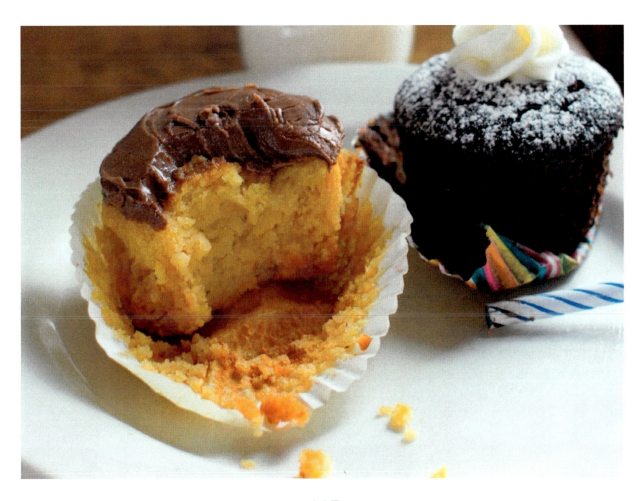

Orange Cream Frosting
Frosts 12 Cupcakes

1/4 C	Palm Shortening
1/4 C	Cooked Orange Yam, skinned
1 Med	Orange, *with* Skin, Deseeded
1/3 C	Erythritol *or* Powdered Sugar
1 t	Vanilla Extract
1/2 t	Almond Extract
	Pinch of Sea Salt
	Stevia drops to taste

Combine all the ingredients in your 4 C Food Processor and Blend until smooth.

TIP: Use a sweet, thinner skinned Orange.

TIP: The orange Yam or yellow Sweet Potato works equally as well. Simply set on a cookie sheet and bake at 325 for an hour or more until soft. Or, of course use your microwave. You or your dog can eat the rest for lunch.

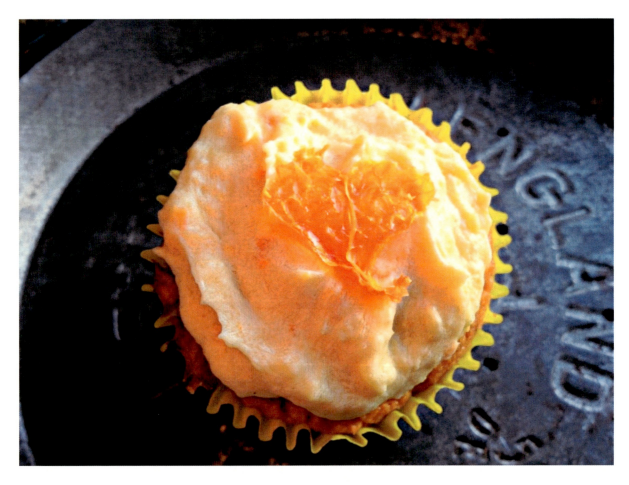

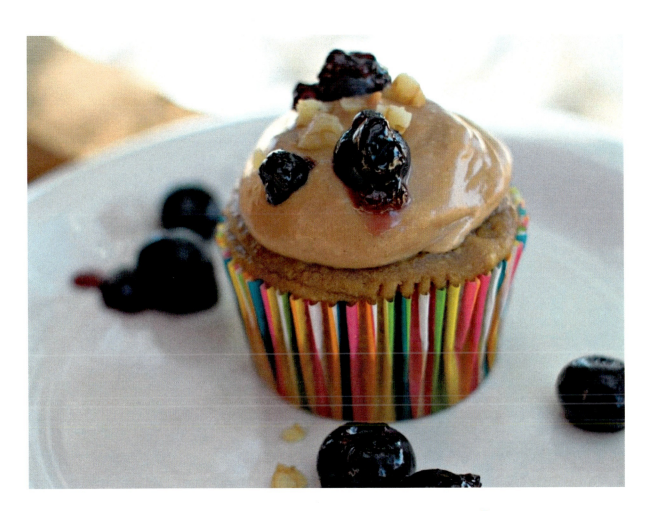

Peanut Butter Frosting
Frosts 12 Cupcakes

2/3 C	Soft Butter *or* Palm Shortening
1/3 C	Smooth Peanut Butter
1/3 C	Maple Syrup
3 T	Cooked Sweet Potato *or* 1T Arrowroot
2 t	Vanilla Extract
	Pinch of Salt (amount depends upon whether your Butter and Peanut Butter are salted or unsalted)
	Stevia drops to taste

Blend everything together in your 4 Cup Food Processor until smooth.

NOTE: Buy Valencia or Jungle Peanut Butter (see resources) to stay clear of very dangerous fungus residues.

Sweet or Coconut Whipped Cream

1 ½ C	Heavy Whipping Cream *or* the 'Chilled' thick Cream from a can of Coconut Milk.
2 T	Erythritol
1 t	Vanilla Extract (optional)

Beat together with your Hand Held Mixer until thick and fluffy and soft peaks form.

White Chocolate Cream

4 T	Chopped White Chocolate
1 C	Heavy Cream
1/2 t	Vanilla Extract

Melt the White Chocolate in the Heavy Cream, add the Vanilla and stir to combine. Chill 'til very cold and whip to soft peaks with your Hand Held Mixer.

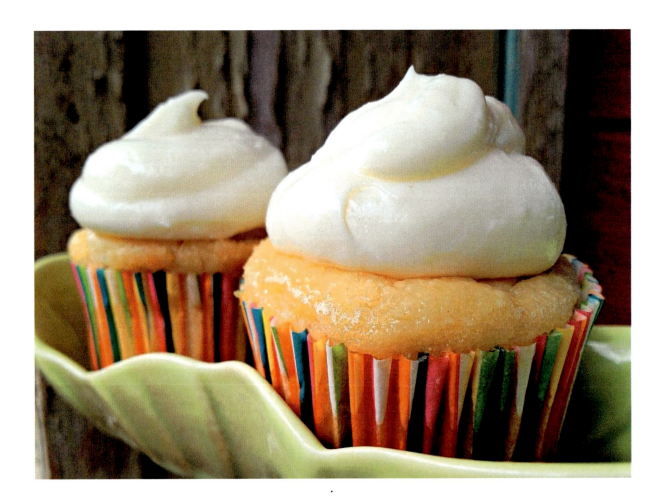

7 Minute Meringue Frosting
Frosts 12 Cupcakes

1 LG	Egg White
1/3 C	Erythritol *or* Evaporated Cane Sugar
2 T	Honey
1 ½ T	Water
1/8 t	Cream of Tartar
1/8 t	Sea Salt
1 t	Vanilla Extract
1/2 t	Almond Extract

Combine all the ingredients except the Extracts in a Double Boiler (or use a Tall Stainless Bowl set on a pan of Boiling Water; don't let the bottom of the pan touch the water).

Beat with your Hand Held Mixer for 6 minutes, it will become light and creamy and triple in size.

Remove the bowl from the heat, add the Extracts and Guar, if using, and continue to beat another minute.

TIP: Add 1/8 t Guar Gum if you plan to freeze these.

NOTE: Remember, if you use Erythritol, it will be a little crunchy!

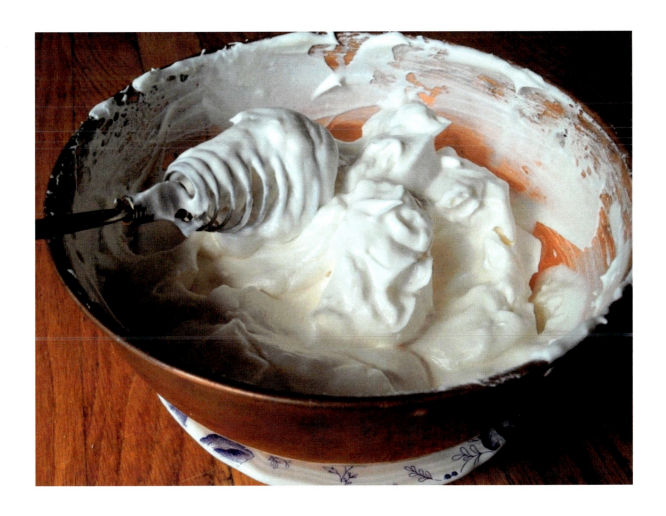

Sweet Sauces

Dark Coconut Palm Caramel Sauce

1 ½ C	Coconut Palm Sugar
6 T	Water
2 T	Butter

Combine ingredients in a small saucepan and stir over medium heat until sugar is dissolved. Cover and allow to boil, without stirring, for about 3 minutes. The steam will wash down the sides of the pan. Uncover and boil another few minutes. The Caramel Sauce will thicken as it cools.

If you wish to use a candy thermometer allow it to reach 238 degrees, the softball stage.

Easy Chocolate Sauce

2 oz	Dark Chocolate
1/2 C	Erythritol *or* Evaporated Cane *or* Palm Sugar
1/3 C	Warm Water *or* Coffee *or* 6 T Heavy Cream *or* Coconut Milk
1 t	Vanilla Extract
	Pinch of Sea Salt

Blend this up in your blender until smooth! Or, if you prefer, heat and stir in a small pan on the stove, adding more liquid as needed.

INGREDIENT RESOURCES

If you don't order online, good whole foods store will also carry these ingredients

ALMOND PRODUCTS
honeyville.com
sunorganicfarm.com

ARROWROOT & BAKING POWDER
bobsredmill.com

CHOCOLATE PRODUCTS
dagobachocolate.com
sunspire.com
navitasnaturals.com

COCONUT PRODUCTS
nutiva.com
tropicaltraditions.com
wildernessfamilynaturals.com

ERYTHRITOL
nowfoods.com
swansons.com
organiczero.com

EXTRACTS
flavorganics.com
mountainroseherbs.com

FREEZE DRIED FRUITS
nuts.com
wildernessfamilynaturals.com
therawfoodworld.com
organicfruitsandnuts.com

HONEY
reallyrawhoney.com

MAPLE SYRUP
maplesource.com

DRIED EGGS
amazon.com
roseacresfarms.com

NUTS
nuts.com
organicfruitsandnuts.com
therawfoodworld.com
sunfood.com (Jungle Peanut Butter)
traderjoes.com (Valencia Peanut Butter)

ORGANIC PRODUCE
organicfruitsandnuts.com
localharvest.org
wholefoodsmarket.com

SALT
mountainroseherbs.com
livesuperfoods.com

SHORTENING
spectrumorganics.com

STEVIA
sweetleaf.com
nowfoods.com

SWEETENERS
wholesomesweeteners.com
jarrow.com (Lo Han Sweet)
bodyecology.com (Stevia/Lakanto)

BAKING GOODS
williamsonoma.com

FOOD PROCESSORS/BLENDER
cuisinart.com
kitchenaid.com
vitamix.ocm

VARIETY
amazon.com
azurestandard.com
traderjoes.com
shoporganic.com

RESOURCES

BOOKS

Wheat Belly by Dr. William Davis
Grain Brain by Dr. David Perlmutter
Gut and Psychology Syndrome by Dr. Natasha Campbell
Body Ecology Diet by Donna Gates
Rainbow Green Live Food Cuisine by Dr. Gabrielle Cousens
Ultra Metabolism by Dr. Mark Hyman
Breaking the Vicious Cycle by Elain Gottschall
Why We Get Fat and What to do About It by Gary Taubes
Nutrition and Physical Degeneration by Dr. Weston A. Price
Nourishing Traditions by Sally Fallon and Mary Enig
Eat Fat, Lose Fat by Dr. Mary Enig
ADHD-the Great Misdiagnosis by Julian Stewart Haber
The Paleo Solution by Robb Wolf
Know Your Fats by Dr. Mary G. Enig
This Ain't Normal Folks by Joel Salatin
In Defense of Food by Michael Pollan
The Hundred Year Lie by Randolph Fitzgerald

WEBSITES and BLOGS

Mercola.com
BodyEcology.com
LocalHarvest.com
RawFoodWorld.com
WestonAPrice.org
DoctorYourself.com
WHFoods.org
NaturalNews.com
MarksDailyApple.com

My NEW book is now available!

The Ultimate Grain Free Cookbook:
Sugar-Free, Starch-Free, Whole Food Recipes from my California Country Kitchen

Visit our website for all the details
www.californiacountrygal.com

You can also find us here...

facebook	instagram	pinterest	twitter
calcountrygal	californiacountrygal	calcountrygal	calcountrygal

Please try our Grain & Starch Free Baking Mixes at

CaliforniaCountryGal.com

Thank you *always* for your support!

Made in the USA
Columbia, SC
22 November 2021

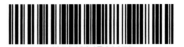